09 1/10/20 0

D0201098

MEMORY LESSONS

MEMORY LESSONS

A Doctor's Story

JERALD WINAKUR

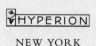

NEW YORK

"Lay Back the Darkness", from *Lay Back the
Darkness: Poems* by Edward Hirsch, copyright © 2003
by Edward Hirsch. Used by permission of
Alfred A. Knopf, a division of Random House, Inc.

Library of Congress Cataloging-in-Publication Data
is available upon request.

ISBN 978-1-4013-0302-0

Hyperion books are available for special promotions,
premiums, or corporate training. For details contact Michael
Rentas, Proprietary Markets, Hyperion, 77 West 66th Street,
12th floor,
New York, New York 10023,
or call 212-456-0133.

Book design by Jennifer Ann Daddio

FIRST EDITION

1   3   5   7   9   10   8   6   4   2

For My Mother and Father

FRANCES AND LEONARD WINAKUR

CREED

If you ask me what I believe in,

it is the body of the ninety year old
straining to stand upright, each vertebra
a testament, each muscle a miracle.

It is the shape of her head,
a sculpture the artist
has been working on for centuries,

the skull visible
under the veil of skin,
and if you ask me for a sermon

I will give you that skin,
every wrinkle a parable.
If you insist upon sacrament

I say take her hand in yours:
it is the only way to save yourself.
Fold your flesh into her bones

until you do not have to ask me anymore
what to believe in.
It is the body

the body,

Amen.

—LEE ROBINSON

MEMORY LESSONS

INTRODUCTION

I am the son of an old, old man. If my father heard me refer to him this way, his feelings would be hurt. In his head he is still young—he cannot remember from one minute to the next that he can't lift himself from a chair and needs the assistance of a strong arm and a walker to get from the living room to his bedroom. Up and balanced on his unsteady legs, he will say: *What happened? What's wrong with me?*

He wouldn't understand that when I refer to him as one of the "oldest old" I am using a gerontological term, a term of art that designates the fastest-growing demographic segment of American society, those over eighty-five. Caring for people like my father is my art, and I have spent my life—the last thirty-plus years of it—in the service of my patients as an internist and geriatrician.

This is a book about my life as a doctor, as the son of an "old, old" man, and as the surrogate son for many of my patients over the years. I think of this book as part memoir, part manifesto. It is about my life in medicine, my evolution as a doctor of the oldest old and the changes I have witnessed in my profession. At the center of this story is my family—my parents, especially my father. I am who I am today in good measure because of him.

In 2005 I wrote an essay titled "What Are We Going To Do With Dad?" This piece described what it is like, from my vantage point as a doctor specializing in geriatrics, to witness my father's descent into disability and dementia, my mother by his side. The piece was first published in *Health Affairs*, a health policy journal. An excerpt appeared in the *Washington Post,* and from there it was syndicated in papers across the country. I had intended this essay to add to the national conversation Americans must have about how we will deal with our impending flood of elders as my generation ages. I was not expecting the response: calls for my appearance on NPR's *The Diane Rehm Show* and Terry Gross's *Fresh Air*, interviews on local radio and television shows in my hometown, invitations to speak at national gatherings of healthcare providers, to present grand rounds at academic medical centers, to author a column on aging and elder care.

But most of all, I was not prepared for the e-mails and letters—thousands of them—I have received from around the country and the world. I have spent my years as a doctor solving problems—social as well as medical—that arise in my patients, one at a time, in my office examination and consultation rooms or at their bedsides in hospitals and nursing homes. Suddenly I was receiving hundreds of messages a day: pleas for help and advice for an elder parent or an ill spouse; heartbreaking stories of neglect and loneliness; disappointing encounters with medical professionals; nightmarish tales of end-of-life suffering; deep expressions of guilt by children living far from home; requests for appointments by elders living in other states; and advice on how to die quickly and painlessly. I brought up my e-mail each day with a feeling of inadequacy and sometimes even dread.

I am not a research scientist, a policy wonk, or a philosopher. I am not a sage or a guru. I am only a doctor, a clinical internist and geriatrician, one who has done his best to listen carefully to each patient in turn and confront every problem with a reasonable fund of knowledge, a modicum of common sense, and a large dose of honesty.

———

Today there are 4.5 million people in our country among the "oldest old." Only one in twenty is fully mobile. Fifty percent are cognitively impaired. Perhaps your parents are among these. Or your spouse. Or maybe even you yourself.

By 2030 there will be seventy-two million people in America over sixty-five and almost ten million of them will be among our "oldest old." By 2050 this fastest growing demographic segment of our society—those over eighty-five—will quadruple today's numbers.

I wish I were bold enough or smart enough to write a book titled *The Ten Things You Must Know to Help Your Parents Through Old Age . . . And You Through Your Own.* This is not that book.

We all search for answers; we all want to do the "right thing" for our parents, for the sake of our life partners and ourselves, and, of course, for the sake of our own children. And yet we often don't know what that "right thing" is. I certainly don't pretend to have all the answers.

Every family travels its own path with loved ones at life's end and discovers that at this destination what remains is only memory. When that is gone, as it is with my father, it falls to me, the son, to gather the threads of our old life, weave them into the tangle of our present circumstances, and make some sense of it all. It is my hope that this book, my family's story, my patients' stories, will enlighten this journey.

So I find that I am writing this book for two reasons. I am searching my past—as a son and as a doctor—in an attempt to come to terms with my father's and my mother's aging process and impending demise, knowing full well that I am next in line. And while I say that this is not an instruction manual for aging, I am also writing it in the hope that these stories will, in the end, resonate with you and your loved ones. Perhaps you will glimpse in the splintered light of these words, filtered through my personal prism, a glimmer of your own truth.

ONE

On my twelfth birthday—the year was 1960—my father gave me a copy of Roger Tory Peterson's *A Field Guide to the Birds of Eastern North America*. All my young life he had told me stories of his boyhood in the Baltimore of the 1920s, how he had fallen in love with birds, trekked through the woods following each new one until he could sneak up for a close look. He had no field guide then, no binoculars. After every woodland foray, after he committed to memory the shape of each bill and wing, the pattern of colors and spots, the flight and foraging behaviors, he ran to the Enoch Pratt Free Library and looked up each bird in turn. In this way he came to know the Baltimore oriole, the scarlet tanager, the rufous-sided towhee, and all the birds that inhabited the outskirts of the city in which he was born.

I had never heard of Roger Tory Peterson until that day when my father gave me this field guide. Over my lifetime I came to know Peterson through his work, his paintings, and his writings. He is, in some ways, a lot like my own father. He was born in Jamestown, New York, in 1908, of immigrant parents. He wasn't very good at schoolwork—"not college material," as he described himself—and he followed his passion for drawing and painting birds throughout his life. His real love was always bird portraiture. He wanted his legacies to hang on the walls of museums, like John James Audubon's or Louis Agassiz Fuertes'. In an interview he said he didn't have much time to pursue his paintings. "I'm known for the guides," he said, "and everybody wants more and more." He stayed extremely busy. He traveled to Antarctica seventeen times, saw 4,500 species of birds all over the world. There are over fifty titles in his Field Guide series.

On my twelfth birthday my father and I were sitting together on the back stoop of our home on Green Meadow Parkway in northwest Baltimore. I was pouting because a new baseball glove, not a field guide, was the present I had hoped for. I did not then share my father's interest in birds or the natural world. I was halfheartedly thumbing through the pages until I was startled by Peterson's rendering of an indigo bunting. The bird jumped off the page at me. It was such a vivid illustration, an animated, almost otherworldly electric blue.

"Have you ever seen an indigo bunting?" I asked my father.

"Sure," he said. "There are lots of them around here this time of year."

He was staring across our lawn to the weed-choked berm across the alleyway.

"There's one now," he said.

"Where?" My head was out of the book and I was searching the profusion of early wildflowers, but I didn't see the bird.

"Try these." He reached behind and offered up his Army-issued binoculars that had sat, heretofore, on the top shelf of his bedroom closet, a place I was forbidden to explore. "Happy birthday, Jerry-boy," he said.

He passed those binoculars into my hands and looked into my face. I remember taking the glasses from him and putting them up to my eyes. The bunting, in perfect light, came into focus and was the most beautiful thing I had ever seen in my young life.

Is it possible that one day I will forget this sight?

My father has forgotten almost all he ever knew about birds. Most days he forgets I am his son. He is always pleased to see me, although much of the time he thinks I am his brother or some old friend whose name he can't remember. At the end of our visits he always says, "You ought to come around more often," even if I last left only hours before.

At eighty-six, my father is a member of the fastest-growing demographic segment of American society, the "oldest old." Almost half of all people my father's age suffer from some degree of cognitive impairment, or dementia, whether recognized or not by their families. Those between seventy-five and eighty-four—my mother falls into this category—are the "old old." Seniors over sixty-five yet younger than seventy-five are, in this schema, referred to as the "old," a designation I myself—along with millions of baby boomers—am rapidly approaching.

After each visit with my father, if he is still awake, I say, "I love you, Dad."

And it is always a surprise when he answers, "I love you, too," because this is something my father could never bring himself to say when I was his twelve-year-old son or even his fifty-year-old son. But now that I am almost sixty and he is close to ninety, he has lost whatever inhibitions, whatever stern governor, had prevented him from openly expressing his affection for me and my brother during the years when he was our father undiminished. This is one gift his progressive dementia has given us.

Each indigo bunting remembers the migratory route back to his home ground—flown in a single night's mighty effort each spring from the Yucatán Peninsula across the treeless black void of the Gulf of Mexico—guided by a map of the heavenly constellations imprinted on his brain. When land is at last in sight, he recognizes the coastline and river systems at the edge of the continent. On his final approach he recalls specific stands of sheltering live oaks, breathes in the smells of the local marsh. He has found his way home and at dawn he whistles a song he heard his father sing years before. Without these memories, he is lost.

We are all growing old. This is not a revelation, although it often tends to be a rude awakening. This is what people do, after all, what all living creatures have done since the first self-replicating strand of nucleic acid made its initial—inevitable—copying error. Human cells have the ability to divide only a certain number of times before the ink of the instruction manual filed in the nucleus begins to smear and the metabolic machinery begins to sputter and rust. It is of interest but of no solace that the only mature adult cells which continue to divide endlessly and ceaselessly in tissue culture are cancer cells. This phenomenon is called "immortality in culture," a cruel joke by the cell biologists who first described this behavior. There is no immortality in *our* culture, deny it as we may.

At fifty-eight years old, the father of two daughters, one still in grad school, I am on the leading edge of a demographic tsunami, the baby boomers. Increasingly we will find ourselves sandwiched between the competing needs of our aging parents and our own children. Although my generation—for the most part—still has our wits about us, we also, like my dad, forget or at least refuse to admit that we are aging. Not only do we do everything we can to look young and feel young, but we do our level best to avoid talking about aging and death. Seventy-five percent of Americans have not communicated to anyone—not even their closest loved ones—their own wishes about how they want to die. Yet despite our massive national denial, the demographic reality of a vast inland sea of elders will soon overwhelm the weakened levees of our health-care system.

I don't know if my father will be alive when I type the last words of this book or when it comes fresh and crisp from the publisher. If he is alive, I will bring him a copy and place it in his hands. If his dementia hasn't progressed much—wishful thinking on my part, I know—and if he is having a good day, he will take this book and leaf through it. My father, who never graduated from high school, has always loved to read; a book is always perched on his nightstand or beside him when he falls asleep. His room, now bereft of his marriage bed, accommodates a hospital bed, commode chair, wheelchair, and a walker. His crowded bookcases still stand against one wall, overflowing with novels, biographies, histories, and art books. Even now my father is always holding a book, even now when his mind is unable to carry a thought from one page to the next.

When my father was the age I am now, he had his first heart attack. After surviving almost five years in the Army Air Corps during World War II, building a small business and then losing it, raising two sons, after rediscovering his passion for art and painting dozens of vibrant canvases, my father began his slow decline. At sixty-five, the year he qualified for Medicare, he had another big heart attack that left him with poor cardiac function. Then, when he was seventy-five, he developed prostate cancer and endured a series of radiation treatments. At eighty-one he became short of breath. His doctor admitted him to the hospital with congestive heart failure.

At first he seemed to be responding to the treatment, the diuretics aimed at reducing his fluid burden, the supplemental oxygen. But the disruptive rhythm of the hospital environment, the strange faces, the constant blood testing, and the trips back and forth to radiology began to overwhelm him. Within two days he became paranoid and delusional. He was unable to sleep or eat. He could not separate his dreams from reality. The demons of his gathering delirium circled him like a pack of wolves, stalked his fragile connection to what was real—his home, his wife, his sons. He lashed out at the demons, those only trying to provide his care, who came bearing sustenance.

"Get away from me!" he shouted. "Take me home. Please take me home!" He grew combative and had to be subdued, at first with chemicals and then with physical restraints for his own protection and that of his caregivers.

The wolves had laid him bare.

———

I never thought my father would reach the age of eighty-six. Until relatively recently—the last half-century in America—in the entire history of man on earth, very few have lived to this age. Indeed, the vast majority of all people who have ever lived past the age of eighty are alive today. In my years as a physician I have watched as our modern medical-industrial complex has evolved one life-prolonging medication and procedure after another—from antibiotics to kidney transplants to coronary stents to cholesterol-lowering drugs—each advance contributing to the longevity of our species. And still, all too often, as I look around at those to whom I minister, I find that the quality of the life many of us lead in our old, old years leaves much to be desired.

My father has been at home now for over five years since his last hospital stay. So far, through the determination of my aging, almost blind mother, the help of my brother, and the daily assistance of a dedicated home health aide, I have been able to keep the promise I made to myself when my father was last discharged: no more hospital stays. I will try—my family is trying—to keep him home until the sounds of his breathing cease, his body is finally at rest, and his mind is at peace in the bedroom where he has slept almost every night these past twenty-seven years. I hope I will be there by his side.

Although I am a doctor, please do not believe for a minute that I have all the answers to the myriad problems that will ambush my family as we struggle each and every day with my father and then, too soon, my mother at life's end. These will be difficult times and we will muddle through them together as so many families have done. I may be a geriatrician, but coming to grips with the ravages and the realities of the aging process in my father has been no easier for me than for anyone. Even though I have the experience to know what is coming, the training to describe in detail the pathologic progression of his disease, the medical vocabulary to document each step of his demise, I am powerless to prevent any of it. The best I can do to assuage my sadness is to recognize the sublime that sometimes occurs in the midst of days when my first impulse might be to retreat. Even in these heartbreaking times I have often learned valuable lessons I hope to pass on.

When I think about my father's brain, I see it the way a doctor does: a radiologist staring at an MRI scan or a pathologist peering through a microscope at a thin slice of tissue fixed to a slide. The radiologist sees generalized atrophy of brain substance, shrunken cortical hemispheres, and excess water where once vital neural connections existed. The pathologist sees a loss of neurons—the functional brain tissue itself—and a sharp decline in the electrochemical or synaptic junctions between the cells, where the complex interpretations of the outside world are analyzed and where memories are stored. And throughout the slide, throughout my father's brain, are the plaques of dysfunctional cells, the tangles and knots of interrupted connections, the detritus of a dying organ.

There is great mystery here. At times I sense the chaos just beneath the surface of his thoughts and actions, his constant fight to maintain some connection to a reality mixed up with dream and nightmare. He is agitated and frightened as he tries to make sense of a life cast adrift from a past. I can only watch, can only cry out from a distant shore as his mind—muddled and lost—tries to work through the same set of conundrums each day:

Is this silver-haired woman really my wife? Frances is young and beautiful, with long raven hair. Is this really my home? Where is the kitchen? It was always downstairs and now there are no stairs, so how can I get there? And this man who says he is my son—I recognize him, I like him, even. But he is too old to be my son. Maybe I am his son? Or maybe he is my brother? But I think that my brothers are both dead—I remember that someone told me they are dead. I'm afraid to ask. Why is my face wet? I don't know why my face is wet . . . and why can't I get up by myself from this chair? What's wrong with me? Am I really old so soon? I just sat down, didn't I? How could I be old?

It's a mystery because on other days he will turn to me and say: "Remember those big rock we used to catch off Thomas Point Light?" And we will have a grand reminiscence about those times: rising at 4 A.M., driving through the deserted streets of our neighborhood and onto the beltway to Glen Burnie, stopping for a bacon and egg breakfast at the White Coffee Pot, loading our gear and five-horsepower Johnson outboard into the rented rowboat docked on the South River, yanking the starter cord, hearing the engine roar to life, smelling the fumes, plying our way out to the river's mouth toward the flashing beacon of the lighthouse just as dawn breaks to the cries of gulls and the sight of diving ospreys; crushing up the clamshell bait and spooning it overboard, hoping to attract a school of striped bass that we of the Chesapeake call "rock"; drifting our baited hooks out into the tide, into our stream of chum, waiting now for that first strike. My father will remember it all. And then nothing.

He was my captain then and now I am his. His son, the geriatrician, who comes to fill some of his empty hours with conversation, comes to fill his daily pill containers, who adds a tad more diuretic when he is short of breath, who tries something new at night to ease the terrors—and takes it away again when it just seems to make things worse. I am the son who tries, mostly in vain, to crank his memory over one more time, jump-start it in the hope that we can skim across the water together for just one more trip out to the lighthouse.

TWO

I 'm ten years older now than my dad was that April night in 1968 when, after the assassination of Martin Luther King, Jr., my father's business was lost. Despite this national tragedy, this murder of a great man, our country was ultimately changed for the better. My father, an average man caught up in these tumultuous times, was also changed, but he was never able to recover from the losses he suffered in the civil unrest of those days.

All of us—my father, mother, my younger brother, and I—had devoted our lives to growing a family business, a pawnshop located at the corner of North Avenue and Pulaski Street in Baltimore. It was our small fragment of the American Dream and in a matter of hours it was destroyed, a victim of those angry times.

I often think about those years my family worked together in that store, wondering what it would be like if I had taken the pawnshop over from my father as he did when his own father died of pneumonia at the age of fifty, just at the start of the Great Depression.

But this was not what my father wanted for me. In 1965 I was a freshman at Bucknell University. In the middle of my first semester I ended up in the hospital with pneumonia and missed two weeks of classes. I was behind in my work, afraid I might fail organic chemistry. I was homesick and depressed. My parents drove up to Lewisburg on a Sunday, their only day off. They picked me up from my dorm, drove me to a park on the banks of the Susquehanna River. My father and I walked along the water's edge. It was autumn; the leaves were turning and dropping. We didn't speak; the river was running strong and would have drowned out our voices anyway. He had brought our binoculars and pointed into the low branches of a sycamore hanging over the water. I saw my first yellowthroat, but there was no thrill in it for me that day.

My parents made sure I had a good solid meal at a restaurant, fried chicken and mashed potatoes. My mother would turn to me every hour or so and ask, "Are you okay, now?"

"Sure," I said. "I'm fine." My father said nothing.

They stayed with me until the sun was setting; they would drive back to Baltimore in the dark.

At the men's quad we lingered over our good-byes. My parents were about to pull away. I hung on to the car, leaning in through my mother's window.

"Wait," I said. "I want to come home."

"But this semester," my mother said. "Your education . . ."

"I'll work with Dad in the pawnshop," I said.

My father looked across my mother at me. "You're staying here."

"But, Dad, I don't think I can do this . . ."

"You're staying here." And he rolled up the window and drove away.

Years later my mother told me that he cried like a child on the three-hour drive home.

I was ten when my father was forced to move the pawnshop after the City of Baltimore took the old store by eminent domain for the University of Maryland School of Medicine. The new Star Loan Office on North Avenue and Pulaski Street had been a typical brick Baltimore row house, one with white-marbled steps out front. My father completely gutted it on the inside. The new store was a knockout: high-ceilinged, with lighted showcases overflowing with rings and watches that my mother had cleaned and polished, glass-fronted cabinets packed with radios, cameras, and TVs, racks of suits and leather coats. The neon sign hanging over the door blinked: STAR LOANS—ON ANYTHING OF VALUE.

I was proud to work there after school and on Saturdays. In this mostly residential neighborhood, there wasn't another store for blocks where a person could run in and buy a pair of pants, or shoes, or a transistor radio. And cheap.

Our neighbors seemed happy to have us there. My dad always cashed their payroll checks for free. How many times did I see him loan money on a suit with moth holes, or a tinny-sounding radio, just because he knew the customer needed a few dollars to tide him over until his next check came in?

When I think back on it now, it's hard to believe that my father ever made any money in that business. If he loaned someone three dollars on a pair of shoes, he could charge, by law, only twenty-five cents if the item was redeemed within thirty days. For twenty-five cents a month, he documented and described the item in a ledger, made a pawn ticket, filed a police report. The shoes were bagged and labeled, carried upstairs and stored, then down *again* when the shoes were redeemed. For twenty-five cents.

I realized even as a youngster—and I will never forget—how we were perceived by the larger world: money-mongering shylocks, usurious predators, partners with common criminals. My father was ashamed of this image and still is. On the rare occasion that we talk of his years in the business, he gets upset, anxious. "I don't like to think about it," he says. Even now when he is an old man and hasn't set foot in a pawnshop in decades, he is ashamed.

My father is an honest and humble man. He handled thousands

of pieces of jewelry, yet never wore a ring. Nothing but an old, out-of-pawn Bulova watch that wasn't even gold.

For years I sat on a stool next to the yellow Formica counter where he assessed every item as it came in for pawn, watched him meticulously complete the required police report: make, model, serial number, description. I watched as he drew pictures of each jewelry piece, identifying the pattern of stones, the size and color of each one. Each drawing, I remember thinking back then, was a small gem in itself.

When my father was in junior high, a teacher sent home a note to his widowed mother. She beat him before opening it, figuring he'd gotten himself into trouble. Granny, an illiterate and frightened woman from the shtetls of Eastern Europe, didn't need any more trouble. This teacher had recommended my father transfer to a special school for the arts. My father loved to draw, had a real talent for it. His mother, after he read the letter to her, tore it up, dropped it on the ground in front of him, and walked away.

I remember the first time my father told me that story.

"Weren't you mad at Granny?" I asked. "That was so mean of her!"

"She didn't know any better," he said. "She was struggling to keep her family going. We were all struggling."

Granny ended up in a nursing facility after a series of strokes. The home was an old white clapboard house off Reisterstown Road. The lawn had been turned into a graveled parking lot and my father and I pulled into it every Sunday afternoon for the few years before she died. I dreaded these—my first nursing home visits. Granny sat staring, oblivious to everything around her, constantly picking, picking at a huge callus on her hand.

Mom, it's me, Len . . . Can you hear me, Mom? . . . Jerry, come over here so she can see you . . . Give her a kiss . . . Mom, it's my son, Jerry. Mom, can you hear what I'm saying to you? We're going to take you home soon . . . Mom, can you hear me?

Leaving, we'd climb into the old green DeSoto. My father sat quietly for a bit, behind the steering wheel. And then he began to cry. I sat next to him on the front seat and patted him on the shoulder. "I'm okay. I'll be all right," he said.

But he wasn't. When Granny died, he lapsed into a depression for months, though he never missed a day of his long workweek. I often heard him crying at night, sitting up alone. It was a big secret back then, but I know that my mother finally convinced him to see a psychiatrist. He went only once. Years later, rocking on the bay off Thomas Point Light, he looked up from trying to untangle a backlash. It was a real mess, and while he was sidelined, I was catching one rock after another.

"You know why I never went back to see that psychiatrist? Do you know what he said to me about your granny? I mean, I talked to the man for an hour, and he says, 'Did you ever think that maybe you didn't like your mother very much?' Imagine him saying that . . . Son of a bitch! Who doesn't love their mother?"

Instead of pursuing his art, at the end of each day in the pawnshop my father folded up his drawings on the police sheets and dropped them off at the precinct office. A few times a year the detectives came in to claim an item that had been reported stolen. My father turned it over without a word, losing whatever he had in it, glad to be rid of the taint. "But it's not your fault," I said to him. "How could you have known?" I was angry for us both back then.

Working beside my father in the pawnshop taught me how to talk to people, to listen, to treat each one with honesty, compassion, and respect. All my doctoring life my patients have benefited from what I learned from my father. "The customer is always right," he told me many times. My father got along with everyone who came in. Most of them were working people from the neighborhood. He knew their names, addressed them as "Mister" or "Sir," even the angry and distrustful ones, those who were drunk or hopped-up, and always the ones who had fallen on hard times. "You can tell when someone needs a break. Give it to them whenever you can," he told me. I spent my teenage years by his side—after school, Saturdays, my summer vacations. But I never tell anyone about these years—not because of how my father ran his business but because of who he became after he lost it.

Terrence Broom was one of those neighborhood characters who came in regularly to the Star Loan Office. Sometimes he was a perfect gentleman. Once I sold him a suit and he was back the next day asking for me by name so that he could buy a pair of shoes as well. But occasionally, especially if he was drinking, he would run short before payday and bring in some item or other for a loan to tide him over. My father no longer remembers Terrence Broom, but I know why he feels anxious at the mention of this name. It has to do with the time Mr. Broom came in to redeem his tape recorder from pawn.

"How are you today, Mr. Broom?" my father said. Mr. Broom only huffed and threw his pawn ticket down on the counter with some bills. My father handed me the ticket, and I ran up the back stairs to the second-floor warehouse area, that windowless, cavernous space where my family's life savings were stored—not in stocks or bonds or gold bars but in racks of suits and topcoats, radios and TVs, rows of console stereos, rifles and trumpets, piles of hand tools, power tools, shoes, work boots, stacks of electric fans and suitcases. Everything in its place: bagged or wrapped, tagged and numbered. I found Mr. Broom's tape recorder in an instant, ran back down the stairs with it, tore the tag off, and handed the package to him. "Thank you, sir," I said.

He turned and stomped out but was back in ten minutes, red-eyed and bellowing that we had lost the microphone.

"You thief," he yelled at my father. "Sonofabitch," he said. I could smell the alcohol on his breath.

My father answered calmly. "We'll make it right, Mr. Broom. Calm down."

I ran back up the stairs, retraced my steps, looked under the racks, behind the shelves. Nothing. Through the insulation of a thousand hanging garments, a wall of bagged shoes, I could still hear Mr. Broom screaming at my father.

I came back empty-handed. Mr. Broom pounded his fist on the counter. My father offered to order a new microphone from the manufacturer, offered him his pick of any tape recorder for sale in the store. Nothing would appease Mr. Broom.

"You crook! You kike!" he hollered.

I backed away. I knew my father kept a gun under the counter. I wanted him to reach for that .38 police special and level it at Mr. Broom's chest. But he just stood there taking each insult, one after the other

Just then a little boy came in waving the microphone. "It was in the alley behind the house, Daddy," he said. "It musta fell out of the bag . . ."

Without a word, Terrence Broom started walking out.

"Aren't you even going to apologize, *Mister* Broom?" I said. I was a cocky teenager with an overwrought sense of justice.

He whirled around and moved toward me. My father stepped between us. Mr. Broom towered over us both. "No need to apologize, sir. Just a misunderstanding. Come back and see us anytime."

I was ashamed of my father then, but at that moment he was still my father and I was his son. The riots changed that between us.

That April night in 1968 we huddled in our house and listened to the radio as the rioting spread uptown toward our store. I thought about the British in the underground during the Blitz. Then we started getting phone calls from the police: "They're looting your store!" they told my father. "Come down!"

My father sat numb, hollow-eyed.

"Dad," I pleaded with him. "Dad, let's go down there, sit in the store with the lights on . . . You've got a gun!"

He shook his head, my father, this man who had survived five years in Europe during World War II. "I can't shoot somebody over stuff . . . and I'm not risking our lives over it," he said. "Let it go." And so we did. My father never recovered.

The day after the riots, my father and I drove down to the pawn-shop. It was dangerous, but we had to see. The protective metal grates had been torn off, the windows smashed, emptied. The inside of the store was just as bad. Not a display case remained intact. Everything had been picked clean, upstairs and down. Thousands upon thou-sands of items, a lifetime of savings—my college education and my brother's, my parents' retirement—were gone. There were a few Na-tional Guardsmen milling around outside, bewildered farm boys from Western Maryland patrolling what to them must have seemed like a third-world country. They had thrown some tear-gas canisters inside after the fact, thinking that might keep people out of the store. The acrid smell burned our lungs. The Guardsmen looked menacing, but they had no ammunition in their guns and everybody knew it. Be-sides, everything was already gone.

Terrence Broom saw us walking away from the pawnshop. He came over and shook my father's hand and told him how sorry he was, that he'd had no part in the looting. He extended his hand to me, but I wouldn't take it. My father said, "Thank you, Mr. Broom," and that was the last time I ever stood on the corner of North Avenue and Pulaski Street.

It has been so long now that it seems as if those years I spent in the pawnshop at my father's side were someone else's life. My anger is gone. I have only empathy for all those people who struggled in that neighborhood. I couldn't have—almost didn't survive life there. Yet sometimes I wonder how I have survived the life I have led: days at a stretch of sleepless nights; the constant worry over whether or not I did the right thing, made the right call; all the bad news I've had to deliver, all the deathbeds I have stood beside. I understand my father better now because of this. It took me a long time—too long—to really understand.

After the riots, my father just couldn't get himself together. In no time he used up the little savings he had. He mourned his business, his lack of education. The insurance companies, the legal system, and the city turned their backs on him and hundreds like him. There was no coverage, no reparations, not even an apology. His family and friends abandoned him, worried that they might end up having to give him a handout. I remember one aunt saying to another, "He'll be okay. He must have stole plenty."

I finished college and then medical school on scholarships and loans while my father worked a series of dead-end jobs just to put food on the table. My parents sold their house and moved to a tiny apartment. Whenever I called home, my father complained about the demeaning work, how tired he was, how he'd be dead soon.

"Dad," I said, "I'm almost finished. I'll have a practice. Things will be fine. You'll see."

And for a while they were. We moved away from Baltimore, first me and then, eventually, my parents, followed by my brother. I set up a practice in San Antonio, worked days and nights and weekends. My mother came to work for me, answered the phones, greeted the patients and got to know them, opened the mail, and ran the business office. For years she took work home with her every night just to be certain that all the books balanced, that all the forms were filled out correctly. She loved keeping busy, being productive, helping her son.

My architect brother designed my medical building, his first big project after he opened his own architectural firm. My father, happy at first, began to paint again.

He devoured art books and taught himself art history. One evening he sat me down in his living room, a book of Paul Gauguin reproductions across his lap. It was open to the mural *D'où Venons Nous? Que Sommes Nous? Où Allons Nous?* My father was fascinated with the painting, its lush blues and greens, its three distinct groupings of people, these questions written boldly on the work. He needed assistance with the translation—his French was limited to a few phrases remembered from his Army Air Corps days when he was stationed in Paris.

We worked through Gauguin's questions together, confirming our translation with another text he had: *Where Do We Come From? What Are We? Where Are We Going?*

"What does he mean?" he asked me. "What's he trying to say?" He continued to study the painting.

Then he pointed to the old woman, obviously sick, on the far left side of the painting, the one who appears resigned to her fate. "That's where we're all going," he said. Then he closed the book.

Once, without his knowledge, I entered one of his oils, *Wild Wren,* in a local contest. It won a prize. I took him to the show where his painting hung in a gallery, a white-and-gold ribbon fluttering from the frame. "I can't believe it," he said over and over.

This good feeling lasted no more than a week. He had rekindled something in himself, but it was not enough to heal a damaged ego, to make up for his failures. To him, to be valued meant being productive. That meant earning a living.

I got him a job in a retail jewelry store run by some people I knew. He left at lunchtime and never went back. I came up with a dozen ideas for a little business but nothing suited.

He refused counseling. He was always angry with me. He never had an encouraging word to say, could never muster a phrase or two of praise for my accomplishments or for my brother's. He found no joy in anything except his grandchildren. Even though he lived just a few short blocks away in the house I bought for him, I found myself avoiding him. He complained that everyone was away all day while he was alone.

One afternoon I visited him unexpectedly. My mother was still at work in my office. He was lying on his bed reading a book.

"What are you doing here?" he said.

"I had a free afternoon," I said. "I thought I'd come by and see how you were doing."

"How do you expect me to be doing? You stole my wife," he said.

I felt my face flush. "Someone has to earn a living in this house. Obviously, it isn't going to be you."

"Get out," he said.

Not long after, I apologized. I pleaded with him, begged him not to spend the rest of his life bemoaning his past.

"Dad, at least take advantage of the years you've got left. Mom likes working in the office. Do the things you've always wanted to do—take some classes, join some art groups. Enjoy your retirement!" He continued to mope, to live a loner's existence.

He had become my bad seed.

Years passed in this way. My father had a couple of heart attacks and then prostate cancer. He had left Baltimore behind, fled the corner of North Avenue and Pulaski Street, but he could not hide from his own mortality. The looting robbed him of his self-confidence; aging and disease stalked his body. One by one, the things he loved to do— gardening, fishing, and finally his art—he was forced to abandon.

My father can no longer take pleasure or solace in putting paint on canvas; he can no longer draw the simplest geometric figure. Now he has lost his memories—the good ones and most of the bad—of those pawnshop years when his boys were growing up, when our family pitched in to try to make a success in that business during those difficult times.

My brother, Michael, and I are now the repository of our father's memories. The scenes and stories of our father's life, his adventures and misadventures, his strivings and triumphs and failures, remain stored—for the moment—deep within the cortical gyri of our own brains. Some of these memories are second-hand—stories our father told us of the life he lived before we were born. Others, like working beside him in the pawnshop and our fishing trips together on the Chesapeake Bay, are more vivid because we lived them with our own senses. Our recollections are, of course, our own interpretations, but this is all we have. Isn't this the way of memory—always open to interpretation?

We cannot go back in this life, only forward. Even when the future is certain only to bring us pain and loss, we cannot retreat into the memories of our past. Still, I look back on those years when my family worked together in the pawnshop. I remember how we helped each other and I decide today, now, not to get too far ahead of myself, not to make too many plans. I will need to pace myself on this journey, rest when I can.

I know my family needs help now, the kind that I can provide as a son and as a doctor. One day, probably sooner than I want to admit to myself, I will need the help of mine as well.

THREE

I n college I was a biology major. *Bios*. Life. But to make it in medical school I had to master the sciences of deconstruction: organic chemistry, biochemistry, quantitative chemistry, physics. In those labs, one could only infer what was happening. The atoms, the molecules, the forces, were invisible.

Back then I preferred to see the thing for itself, the living being. Euglena whipping around the slide. Amoebas rolling along. Yes, I had taken things apart: I slit open a pot-bellied frog from chin to genitals. The same with hamsters and cats. These animals were served up to me on paraffin-filled trays, cold and dead. Still, I could see that a frog was a frog, run my fingers over its green leathery skin. The hamster's thick coat. The cat's furry tail.

But thinking about doing this to another human made me ill. I had nightmares about walking into the human anatomy lab—shrouded corpses on stainless-steel tables, row after row. Pulling off the sheet, looking into that death mask, those opaque eyes. My hands dissecting another's. The sharp smell of formaldehyde, day after day.

In the summer of 1969, a couple of months before I was to begin my first year of medical school at the University of Pennsylvania, I received a letter from the dean asking me to volunteer for an experimental program open to only fifteen students. If I wanted, I would spend my first year seeing real patients on the hospital wards and in the clinics—medical school training that did not traditionally begin until the third year. This "clinical program" was a radical experiment. Only a place like Penn, the oldest medical school established in America and one of the best, had the audacity to try something like this thirty-nine years ago.

I jumped at the chance, knowing I could postpone Gross Anatomy until my second year.

And so, on my first day of medical school, with no knowledge of human anatomy or physiology or pharmacology, I found myself on the wards of one of the largest teaching hospitals in the country.

The ophthalmologist was explaining to a tiny old woman with a shock of white hair how he was going to fix her cataracts. This ninety-year-old had been blind for many years, but someone had finally brought her into the clinic.

"We're going to make an incision under your cornea and remove the lens," he said. I was standing behind him, alternately watching the patient's face and following along on a pocket-sized colored drawing of a cross-section of the eye. She tried to touch his face, but he kept fending off her hands.

"Certainly, we can't make you any worse off than you are now. Vision-wise, that is. Of course, if you get a post-op infection, you may lose the eye." Then he turned and walked out.

She reminded me of my maternal grandmother. I stayed behind and sat down on the bed next to her.

"Do you understand what they're planning to do?" I asked.

She put her hands up to my face. I took off my glasses and closed my eyes as her bony fingers explored me.

"I trust you, Doctor," she said.

"I'm not the doctor," I said. "I'm just a medical student."

"It's going to be all right, Doctor," she said.

She was "just in for a sore throat." That's what she told me several times at the walk-in clinic where I had been assigned. I was supposed to take a complete medical history, do a full physical examination, and then "present" her case to the harried resident who was overseeing a bunch of us students in the clinic that day.

She refused to get undressed and put on a gown.

"I just have a runny nose and a bad sore throat," she said.

"Look, I'm a medical student and I'm supposed to do a complete physical exam," I said. "It can't hurt . . . Maybe we'll uncover something." I knew this was likely a lie. She was young and pretty and looked perfectly healthy.

"Just check my throat or I'm leaving," she said.

I took a deep breath. "Okay." I wondered how I would satisfy the resident.

I knew a little something about eyes by then. Hers seemed fine, maybe a little redness of the conjunctivae. She had a cold, after all. Her left eardrum was pink, and I asked if her ear hurt. "A little," she said.

Her throat was very red and I could see some yellow stuff toward the back, on the left side, covering a raw-looking lump of tissue. Her tonsil, I figured. There was a symmetric lump on the other side of her throat, and I knew everyone has two tonsils. That thing that hangs down in the middle was red and glistening and looked a lot fatter than mine.

I checked her neck for swollen lymph nodes and there were a few tender ones on both sides, under her jaw, and one pretty-good-sized one almost at the bottom of her neck, just below her voice box. That's as far as she would let me go.

"You have tonsillitis," I told her. "And a left inner-ear infection. Let me present your case to the resident, and I'm sure he'll put you on antibiotics and you'll be fine in a few days."

"Thanks, Doctor," she said.

"I'm a medical student," I said.

I presented her case to the resident.

"What about the rest of her physical exam?" he asked me.

"That's all she would let me do."

"You know, doctors get sued every day because they're not thorough." He slammed his pen down in her chart. "Let's look at her." My face burned.

"I'm the resident on-call here in the clinic," he said to her. "Open your mouth," he said. "Ugly. Okay, we'll give you a script for penicillin." He was running his fingers up and down her neck, checking for nodes. "You have to take all of them . . . Whoa, what's this?" He turned to me. "Didn't you feel this?" he said, his hands at the base of her neck, fingers resting above the bones there.

"I told you about the lymph nodes in her neck," I said.

"This isn't a lymph node. This is the thyroid gland, and this"—he grabbed my hand and ran my fingers over the lump I had felt earlier—"is a tumor of the thyroid gland. Probably a cancer. You forget your anatomy already?" he asked.

She looked at me; her eyes filled with tears. She couldn't speak.

"Couldn't it be something other than a cancer?" I asked. "A cyst, maybe?"

"Maybe. We'll know after surgery," he said.

"Miss," he turned to her. "You have to go into the hospital so we can remove this tumor. You are very lucky we found it when we did."

And then to me. "Now you can complete your examination. You never know what else you might find—metastases to the liver, other areas of lymph node involvement. You never know. Do everything to everybody. That way you won't miss anything." Then he left.

I wanted to put my arm around her, tell her it would be all right. But I didn't know any more than she did. I reached over to the shelf and pulled out a couple of tissues and handed them to her.

"I have to do the rest of the exam," I said.

"It's okay," she said.

The house staff was in awe of Dr. Prima, a renowned clinician and diagnostician. The intern whom I was trailing on the way to rounds with Dr. Prima said, "The guy's amazing. He can just look at a patient, lay his hands on them, and figure out what the problem is. It's amazing."

Dr. Prima had never met the patient or seen his chart. I expected the resident to present the case history in typical fashion, but instead he said only, "Dr. Prima, this is Mr. Post."

Dr. Prima extended his hand, and Mr. Post took it a little reluctantly as he studied the doctor in his long billowing white coat.

Dr. Prima did not let go of his hand.

"You smoke cigarettes, don't you?"

The patient coughed a few times. "I'm trying to quit."

"Notice the permanent yellow nicotine stains on Mr. Post's fingers. I suspect you have smoked two packs of cigarettes per day for more than fifty years. Isn't that correct, Mr. Post?"

"Pretty near," he answered.

Dr. Prima still held his hand. Mr. Post was getting restless.

"Notice also the shape of Mr. Post's fingernails. How rounded they are. Notice that the angle the nail makes with the nail bed is obliterated, is now concave. An obtuse angle."

I looked at my own nails. Then at Mr. Post's. His looked like the ends of drumsticks.

"This is called 'clubbing,'" Dr. Prima said. "Nicotine-stained, clubbed fingers are pathognomonic for carcinoma of the lung."

Mr. Post pulled his hand back. He stared at his fingers. "They've been this way forever," he said to Dr. Prima. "Anyway, I'm here because of my heart." He fidgeted on the bed.

"Not forever," Dr. Prima said. "Where is this man's chest X-ray?" he asked the resident.

"It was read as normal, sir," the resident said. "Except for his enlarged heart."

"Get me the films," Dr. Prima said.

The resident looked at the intern, who looked at me. I turned and ran out of the room and down to X-ray. The tech in the file room actually found the films, a small miracle, and I ran back. Dr. Prima hadn't moved. No one had.

Dr. Prima took the film from its jacket and held it up to the light coming in from the window. "There is a 1.5 centimeter nodule behind the heart. The radiologist missed it. All of you missed it. It will be malignant."

The resident, flustered and red-faced, said, "Dr. Prima, what about his heart? Mr. Post has severe aortic valvular disease . . . Wouldn't you like to listen to his murmur?"

"We do not replace aortic valves in patients who will be dead in six months," Dr. Prima said.

We all trailed out of Mr. Post's room. I glanced back at him. He was still staring at his fingers.

As the chief resident explained to me, the purpose of the General Surgery Clinic was to find cases on which the surgical house staff could operate. "It's like panning for gold," he told me.

I walked into an exam room and introduced myself. She was already sitting up on the table. She looked resigned.

"What brings you into the clinic today?" I asked.

"My breast is bad," she said.

" 'Bad'?" I asked.

"You'll see."

I went through the litany of medical history questions that have by now been etched into my brain. Back then I carried them on notepaper folded into one of the pockets of my white coat.

I examined her as she lay on the table, saving her breasts for last. They were very large and I could feel nothing abnormal.

"Where is this 'bad' part?" I asked.

She looked relieved. "You don't feel nothin', then?"

"Sit up for me and raise your arms above your head," I said.

"That's how I always feel it," she said.

I stared at her breasts. There was a small dimpled area just to the outside of her left nipple. I rolled this area between the fingertips of both my hands. I felt a hard irregular lump.

"That's it. I told you it was bad, Doctor."

"I'll get the resident to take a look. I'm just a student."

"I brought a suitcase," she said.

I left her room and presented her case to the chief resident.

"Terrific!" he said.

"I'm not sure this is a cancer." I knew it must be; I just didn't want to admit it to the patient or myself.

"Let's look at her," he said.

He asked her no questions; examined only her breasts.

"You probably have cancer," he said to her.

"I knew it was bad," she said. "I've got my suitcase with me."

"Good. This young doctor here will arrange your admission to the surgical floor. We'll take care of this for you."

"Thank you, Doctor."

"Nice pick-up," he said to me.

"She found it," I said.

The OR nurse knew it was my first time. After I fumbled as she attempted to help me into the surgical gown, after I plunged my hands into all the wrong finger spaces of both latex gloves she held open for me, she said, "Keep your hands clasped to your chest. Don't even think about touching anything on the table." All I could see of her was her stern eyes, and I said, "Yes, ma'am," though somehow I knew she was younger than I.

This was an orthopedic case, the replacement of an old arthritic hip with a new stainless-steel ball on the end of a metal stem. A large man, white-haired at the temples, with a booming voice, was working over a long incision in what I guessed was the patient's outer thigh. The rest of the body was either covered with heavy blue sterile sheets or curtained off completely from the operative field. There was no way to tell that a person was under there.

The nurse guided me to my place next to the surgeon. Another doctor worked across the table from him.

"Remember," she said, "hands clasped against your chest."

"Ah, we have a medical student scrubbed in with us this morning." His voice filled the OR. "I'm Dr. Grayson. That's Dr. Leone." Neither of them looked up from their task, knocking away excess bone with stainless-steel chisels and hammers. "Yes," I said.

They kept working, the scrub nurse handing them various implements as they called for them: saws and screwdrivers, hammers and planes and drills. The surgeons had fancy names for these things, but, to me, they were just tools.

There was a smell like my old wood-burning kit used to give off when I etched my initials into a piece of scrap.

They cut off the top part of the hip bone, moved the new metal stem and ball into place. Dr. Grayson seemed very happy with his work. He spoke to me as he continued to chisel here, drill there.

"What is the name of the cavity, the socket, if you will, that this new hip will fit into?" Then, as an aside to Dr. Leone: "The patient should only last as long as her new prosthesis, right?"

"We won't hold our breath, will we, Chief?" Dr. Leone said. I had not realized until I heard her voice that Dr. Leone was a woman. Then they both laughed.

"Well, what's it called?" Dr. Leone asked me again. I knew the answer. I had studied a schematic drawing that was tacked to the wall over the sink where I had spent ten minutes scrubbing before coming into the operating suite.

"Acetabulum . . . I think," I answered.

"What do you mean 'you think'?" she said. "Don't you remember your anatomy?" She was intent on planing off a section of bone.

"I haven't had anatomy yet," I said. "I'm in a special program . . ."

"Craziness," she said. "I read something about that. This medical school's going to the dogs. Hand me the rongeur again, will you, nurse."

"Well," Dr. Grayson added, "have you ever seen any orthopedic surgery before, son?" The burning smell wafted up from the table as the drill bit into the bone.

"Well, no . . . but I helped my father finish out our club basement." I don't know what made me say this.

Dr. Grayson and Dr. Leone both stopped what they were doing and looked at me.

"Out of my O.R., now!" Dr. Grayson said to me.

"But . . ."

"Now!" he said.

In the hall, I leaned against the wall. I pictured a stainless-steel ax crashing into the side of my head from above. The nurse who had helped me gown and glove came up and winked at me. She still had on her surgical mask. "Don't worry," she said, "they have no idea who you are. And I won't tell them."

"Thanks," I said.

"You're gonna be okay," she said. "One of these days."

For an entire year it was like this. There was such a gap between what I knew and what I needed to know. People were not "patients" to me; they were not "interesting cases" or "fascinating diseases." They were sick, frightened individuals, hoping to be healed. It was with them, not the white-coated medical hierarchy, that I identified. I was as frightened as they were, had no more idea what was in store for them than they did.

There is no longer a first-year "clinical program" at Penn. But the doctor I am today can, in large measure, be traced back to that year of medical school. I have been, since that time, always a patient first, and have viewed the system—with all its flaws in sharp relief—through incredulous, often horrified eyes.

———

Day one of my second year of medical school I walked into the anatomy lab for the first time. Twelve months would pass before I saw another living, breathing patient. I took my place among the nervous, wisecracking first-year students fresh from college. I could hardly remember being that young.

I removed the plastic sheet, then the formaldehyde-soaked linens. My eyes burned a little, but it was not as bad as I had feared. She was an old woman, emaciated and bent, her skin waxen, yellow like my grandmother Bessie's before she died of pancreatic cancer. Just looking at her, I knew she, too, had struggled with cancer in the end. But someone else had made that diagnosis. Someone else had treated her and ultimately failed. Someone who had first steeped himself among the dead before he had confronted the living. Someone I would never be.

I touched her hand and then I began.

FOUR

Be prepared to present Mr. Rivas's case this Friday at 'M and M' conference," the chief resident of Internal Medicine said to me one Monday morning late in my internship year. All my sphincters tightened; I knew what was coming.

"Rivas?" I asked, searching my tired brain for some recollection of this patient, knowing I must have screwed up somewhere along the line if I was being asked to present his case at the monthly Morbidity and Mortality conference. I thought I had remembered each and every foul-up that year, my first one out of medical school, the first year I could legitimately call myself a doctor.

I may have earned my MD degree, but I was not close to being a fully trained physician. Nevertheless, I was the one primarily responsible for the patients under my care in the ERs and clinics, the wards and ICUs in which I had been working. Back then I carried a stack of index cards in my pocket, each one stamped with a patient's name and hospital ID number, filled with my handwritten notes about every one I had seen while assigned to a given hospital service. Instinctively, I reached for these cards and began to shuffle through them.

"Pedro Rivas," the chief resident said. "You saw him about six months ago at 'The Green.' Bad hypertension. He came into the hospital last week in renal failure. He's on the seventh floor."

"I don't remember him at all . . . ," I said.

"Check out his chart and be ready to present his case." He shook his head and walked away.

"The Green." Once, years in the past, "The Green" was a hospital. Now—in 1974—dilapidated, outmoded, and mostly shut down, it housed a twenty-four/seven walk-in "emergency room" that was nothing more than a hallway lined with fifty or so orange plastic bucket chairs. Two seedy exam rooms opened onto this corridor. Sick people, almost all indigent and Spanish-speaking, sat for hours waiting to be seen by one of the two interns assigned to this rotation. The very sick didn't belong here; these folks, if identified, were taken by ambulance to the county teaching hospital far away from this barrio where they lived. Of course, every so often a critically ill patient—unbeknownst to anyone—sat among all the others with routine colds and sore throats, headaches and other minor ailments, waiting his turn.

One morning at 3 A.M. I had finally caught up with the backlog of patients. There was one chart left in the rack, one last name for me to call, one last poor soul asleep, slumped over in his orange seat, his mouth hanging open. I called out his name. He didn't answer. I walked over to him. He was dead. He went straight to the morgue. No "M and M" conference here. After all, he had received no care.

I had, by this point in my internship, completed two of my three required assignments at "The Green," where we worked thirty-six hours on and twelve hours off for three weeks at a time. No senior residents or faculty were available at "The Green." We interns were on our own.

I hated my rotations there. We all did. In those days, "The Green" represented the height of exploitation in an academic training program—exploitation of a population in need of medical care and of the interns sent to provide it.

During my first three-week rotation I was overwhelmed, awash in sick people with whom I could not communicate. Each time I called out (and usually mispronounced) a name—Jimenez, Salazar, Escamilla, Aguilar—I searched desperately for a bilingual LVN (licensed vocational nurse) or RN (registered nurse) or aide to help me, to accompany me and the patient into the exam room so that I might understand the medical history, wherein 80 percent of the stuff of diagnosis lies. But these overworked personnel had other jobs to do and were seldom available.

By my second rotation I was more prepared. I had learned enough rudimentary Spanish to take a limited medical history and do a physical examination: *¿Dónde le duele? ¿Qué clase de dolor es?* Still, I felt I was missing much important information.

I started keeping notes: numbers of patients seen, what percentage spoke Spanish only, their presenting symptoms, the final diagnosis I had come to, those needing treatment in our small eight-bed observation unit down the hall, the ones I actually admitted to the county hospital.

Armed with this information, I set up a meeting with the head administrator of "The Green." I described my predicament, my concerns that I wasn't doing the kind of job I felt I should be doing, my worries that I was missing potentially serious conditions. I argued for the necessity of hiring bilingual personnel to work as translators in the emergency room. The administrator glanced at my data and listened with a half-smile on his face, as if he had heard all of this before.

"Let me ask you this, Doctor: How many more patients do you think you could see during your shift if we provided bilingual translators?"

I tried to control myself. I had just shown this man meticulously collected data demonstrating that I was seeing an average of 150 patients during my thirty-six-hour shift. My partner, the other intern, was doing the same.

"I would see fewer people," I said. "But I wouldn't be practicing veterinary medicine on the patients coming to your hospital!"

"Translators are out of the question then," he snapped.

I left his office, fuming. I sent a letter to the chairman of the Department of Medicine, the head of my training program. I was told—in so many words—to shut up and buck up. I thought about writing a letter to the city's newspaper. But by then I was demoralized; I had just enough energy to get through each day.

I resolved to make the best of it. I remembered my father's words, about his early years in the pawnshop.

I only had six months to go before high school graduation—I wasn't a great student but still, six months and Granny pulled me out of school to go to work in the pawnshop and I never went back . . . So before long I said, "Well, if this is going to be my life, I'm going to make the best of it." Let that be a lesson to you, Jerry-boy . . .

He came through it. He coped. He worked. What was a rotation at "The Green" compared to his life?

I pulled Mr. Rivas's chart out of the rack at the seventh-floor nursing station of the Bexar County Hospital. He had been admitted a few days before with a blood pressure of 280/130. He was only fifty years old. He wasn't a diabetic and hadn't suffered a heart attack or a stroke. I leafed through his lab reports. His kidneys were functioning at only 25 percent of normal; he would soon need dialysis, ultimately a kidney transplant. But why? What had caused his blood pressure to be so high?

The answer was on the next page of lab values. An analysis of a twenty-four-hour urine collection showed that Mr. Rivas had a rare glandular tumor, a pheochromocytoma, benign except in its production of high levels of adrenaline-like substances that cause malignant hypertension. Undiagnosed and untreated long enough, these elevated pressures damage the kidney and ultimately cause strokes, heart attacks, and kidney failure. With proper treatment—identifying and removing this tumor at an early stage—a patient with this condition can be totally cured.

Mr. Rivas had lost that opportunity because of me. The last page in his chart was a photocopy of my ER note six months before, during my first rotation at "The Green." He had come in complaining of a headache and his blood pressure was 220/110. In my note there was no mention that I had asked about other symptoms common to patients with pheos, such as flushing, sweating, and palpitations. Had I failed to ask because I did not know to ask, or because I did not have the Spanish vocabulary to ask?

I had put Mr. Rivas in the observation unit and started him on intravenous medications to lower his pressure. Over the next hours his headache disappeared and his pressure normalized. I then put him on oral medications and watched him for another twelve hours. His pressures remained normal, as did his kidney function. I had not ordered any urine collections.

I did call the Medicine Clinic and twist the secretary's arm to schedule a follow-up visit for Mr. Rivas in just two weeks. The usual wait time for a new patient appointment was several months. I sent Mr. Rivas out of "The Green" with three prescriptions and an appointment at the Medicine Clinic. He did not keep that appointment; he was "lost to follow-up," as doctors practicing in hierarchical settings learn to say. Had he gone to the clinic, some other doctor—hopefully more experienced than I—might have recognized that his hypertension needed further investigation.

I visited Mr. Rivas in his hospital room. His wife and four children, three girls and a young son, sat around his bed watching television. Mr. Rivas was in no distress; his blood pressure was now normal again. He was waiting to have his tumor removed. I re-introduced myself. Neither of us recognized the other. I shook his hand. "*Cuidate,*" I said to him. Take care of yourself.

On the Friday morning of the Morbidity and Mortality conference, I was too tired to be nervous. I hadn't slept the night before because I had been on-call in the cardiac intensive care unit. I was too numbed, too exhausted, to be intimidated by my superiors.

At the conference I presented Mr. Rivas's case, beginning with our encounter at "The Green." Various faculty members in their long white coats stood up and asked me all the questions I had anticipated. Yes, I knew that in patients with sustained hypertension, a tiny minority had a pheo: five hundred to eleven hundred cases per year in a nation—at the time—of twenty to forty million people with high blood pressure. And yes, of course I knew that it was important to look for curable causes of hypertension—even with odds so small. And yes, now my patient was going to need a kidney transplant. Because of me.

"I don't suppose, Doctor," the chairman said at the end of my presentation in front of the white-coated throng, "that you will ever miss this diagnosis again."

What did he want me to say?

And here is the problem with a system of medical education designed to teach through intimidation and guilt: Mr. Rivas was in renal failure because of a flawed system of medical care. Overworked, exhausted interns (called first-year residents today) in under-funded indigent care facilities, who must deal not only with knowledge gaps but major language and cultural barriers, cannot be expected to perform optimally—*especially* in the absence of faculty supervision and oversight. The situation may be better today than it was thirty years ago but not because the medical academy examined and corrected its own deficiencies. If medical care in teaching hospitals has improved (and one recent study still documents a lack of supervision in more than half the errors made by doctors in training), the paradigm shift responsible for this improvement is a direct result of lawsuits brought against these institutions for injuries and deaths attributable to overwhelming resident workloads.

Of course, this system failure was never explored, never mentioned in that "M and M" conference, or in any one I ever attended during the seven years of my medical training.

I write about this now, with the insight and perspective of a long career in medicine, and still I blame myself for missing Mr. Rivas's correct diagnosis. I should have admitted him to the hospital for his high blood pressure—though I was seeing many patients with these blood pressure levels in those days before powerful and effective anti-hypertensive therapies were developed.

There is a great irony here: I would like my former chairman to know that I have tested hundreds of patients' urines over the decades I have been in practice, at a cost to society of untold hundreds of thousands of dollars. I have never seen another case of pheochromo-cytoma. And despite this, I also want him to know that I will continue to search, no matter what the managed care grunts might say, no matter how loud their actuarial screams over "unnecessary laboratory testing"—because it is the right thing to do, the right way to practice medicine.

Each fall I meet with a group of incoming first-year medical students. The first hour of their education is an ethics class presented by the Center for Medical Humanities and Ethics at the University of Texas Health Science Center in San Antonio. They will read and discuss poems by W. H. Auden and W. S. Merwin, essays by Timothy Quill and Atul Gawande, stories by Anton Chekhov and Richard Selzer.

We present them with dramatic cases that highlight the four principles of medical ethics—autonomy, beneficence, nonmalefi-cence, and justice—that will form the basis of their future relation-ships with their patients as well as their interactions with their medical colleagues and the system of medical care and scientific research in America.

We will then tell them the story of Dax Cowart, a former Air Force pilot, who as a young man was severely burned, blinded, and deformed in a freak accident. Realizing the devastating and life-changing extent of his injuries, Dax clearly and unequivocally expressed his desire to re-fuse treatment and be allowed to die. Despite his protests, his wishes were ignored and even though he is alive now, thirty years later, he continues to chastise the medical profession. Today, as an attorney, he fights for patient autonomy in a healthcare system that often forgets who is at the center of each medical encounter.

Together we watch the movie *Wit*. With gathering horror we witness as Professor Vivian Bearing, a scholar enrolled in an experimental chemotherapy protocol for ovarian cancer, devolves from person to specimen in her doctors' zeal to pursue their research interests. We see how our passion as physicians to "find a cure"—our beneficence—is often in conflict with another ideal, nonmaleficence, or as stated in the Hippocratic oath: *First, do no harm.*

We talk about the fourth principle of medical ethics, social or distributive justice. These first-year students will soon be working in an indigent-care county hospital where obesity, diabetes, hypertension, heart disease, and cancer run rampant; a chronically underfunded facility in a state where one in four of its citizens has no health insurance, the highest rate in the nation. The status of health care here has been labeled "Code Red" in a 2006 report, "The Critical Condition of Health Care in Texas." Fiscal problems like these confront all public-based health-care systems in America today.

After the main lecture I meet my small group of twenty or so. I ask them to tell me about their own experiences with doctors, with our health-care system. They relate stories of grandparents who have died, parents who have been ill, the caring doctor who came into the house or the hospital room. Some describe encounters with physicians who were cold or distant or incompetent. Most of these idealistic first-year students want to go into family practice or general internal medicine, pediatrics or geriatrics. They volunteer at the barrio health clinics, travel to the *maquiladoras* just across the border. They go to India and Africa, Mexico and South America to work in remote health facilities during their summers off.

I spend some time talking to these young students about guilt, about how our system of medical education, with its strict hierarchy—much like the military—is more than willing to let the blame for bad outcomes slide down the ranks. The medical profession has its own way of reinforcing guilt. In all my years of training I was never told that I was not expected to be perfect; indeed, over and over I received just the opposite message. Unfortunately, I believe that this attitude—expected perfection in the training and practice of medicine—is toxic, and yet it is alive and well today, perhaps even more so in this litigious age.

Then I tell them my own story, the story of "The Green."

FIVE

My father never wanted me to go to medical school.

In 1967 I had just finished my sophomore year at Bucknell. After my rocky start as a freshman I had gotten myself in gear and I began to do well. I discovered the new field of ecology, and one of my professors noticed me when I took his class in evolutionary biology. This teacher had a grant to study the ecology of rodents in the Arizona desert and he offered me a summer position as his research assistant. I was nineteen years old and had never been on an airplane. I told my professor that I would meet him in Arizona.

I hadn't yet told my father. I'd been home for the summer just a little more than a week and had gone to work with him every day at the pawnshop as I did in those years before he lost the business.

It was close to 10 P.M. on a Saturday night and we had finally gotten out of the store for the day and had stopped at Mandel's on Reisterstown Road for a bite to eat on our way home. I ordered my usual deli special: corned beef on rye with coleslaw and Russian dressing. My father had a bagel and a bowl of matzo ball soup.

"So, Jerry-boy, tell me about college. We've hardly had a chance to talk since you got home."

I knew this was my chance. "I took a course in ecology last semester. I really liked it."

"I read about that," he said. "It's about how living things adapt to their environment . . . something like that anyway," he said.

"That's right, Dad. I'm learning a lot . . ."

"Sounds terrific, Jerry-boy. Maybe you should consider going into that instead of medical school. Be a college professor. If you become a doctor, your life will never be your own. You'll be around sick and dying people all the time . . ."

"Dad," I said, "my ecology professor has offered me a chance to do research with him this summer in Arizona. For two months. I know how you depend on me here at the store . . ."

"You'll be with this professor?"

"I'll stay with him and his family. He's got a research grant and he's paying my airfare and a salary for the summer . . ."

"You like this man?"

"Very much. And he loves to watch birds, knows them all."

"Well, that's it, then," he said. "You're going to Arizona."

Two years later, by the time I had to make my choice between ecology and medicine, the pawnshop was gone. I had already become a caretaker.

In the early years of my practice I knew only two things for certain. I wanted to be a "real" doctor: someone to whom an adult might come with just about any complaint or ailment and get a complete assessment—an accurate diagnosis or at least a working list of possibilities or "differential diagnoses"—along with a plan of action until a definitive answer could be found and a course of treatment was clear. I wanted to be a doctor who would be there by his patient's side through the worst of times. A doctor who would be there, not just around the clock but throughout a lifetime. A real doctor, not a technician.

The second thing I knew for certain is that I never wanted to become an "LMD," an acronym for Local Medical Doctor, a term of derision that some of my mentors reserved for those privately practicing physicians who constantly flub diagnoses, mistreat and abandon their patients and, worst of all, practice fee-for-service medicine. Of course, there is a built-in bias here since the medical scientists who teach young doctors are, for the most part, super-specialists with narrow research interests in their own fields. They do not see vast numbers of patients, if they see patients at all.

Perhaps if I hadn't been a harried resident in my training days, or if I had come from a lineage of doctors, I might have seen through this bias. But I was like a surgical sponge, soaking up knowledge, emulating attitudes, bloodily becoming a doctor. For better or worse, I was determined not to end up an LMD.

Of course, that is exactly what I am today, three decades after completing my residency program. In fact, an LMD is what I have been from the moment my first patient was escorted into the examination room of my first rented office less than a mile from the university hospital where I trained. I don't believe I fit the stereotype my mentors derided, but I have been a real-world doctor and nothing more. There are thousands like me out here, mostly serving our patients well. Like so many of my colleagues, I am proud to have been an LMD all these years, despite the fact that on occasion my faith in my abilities has been shaken.

I met my first wife in medical school. Leslie was one of only seven women admitted to Penn that year in our class of one hundred and fifty. She was lovely and bright and irreverent; I couldn't believe my good fortune that she fell in love with me. We married after our first year of med school. After graduation, we entered the same residency program in San Antonio together, she in pediatrics. One main criterion in choosing our programs was that our respective departments promised to coordinate our on-call schedules so that we would have the same nights and weekends off together. Most of the other residency programs had scoffed at this request. Their message was clear: Your marriage is a footnote to your medical career.

Leslie got pregnant during our third and final year of residency training. She took a week of vacation before giving birth to Betsy, our first daughter. We juggled through the second half of that year—my wife on call at the hospital one night while I stayed home with the baby, the reverse scenario the following night, and all of us home together the third night. That was one of the sweetest years of our married life.

It was my idea to go into private practice together. Leslie was skeptical, worried about the long hours and the stress involved. Together, I thought, we would maintain our enthusiasm and make a success of a joint practice: she caring for the newborns and kiddos, I for the parents and grandparents and eventually her patients when they grew up. How could we fail?

We took two weeks off after finishing our residencies and traveled back East to visit family. When we returned, July 12, 1976—our sixth wedding anniversary—we opened our medical office for business. Within that first year, Emily was born. Between the eighty-hour work weeks, the emergency room summonses, the dozens of phone calls every evening and throughout each night, the weekend on-call schedule—and, of course, raising our kids—we had little time for each other. Our practice, however, was a big success.

During the years we were raising our young family, my great aunt Lena came to San Antonio each winter for a month or so. She was the younger sister of my mother's mother, Grandma Bessie. Bessie was the family matriarch, hard-working, strong, and tender; her love for me was unconditional. Aunt Lena had traveled with Bessie to America in 1909 from their family's shtetl in the Pale of Russian settlement near the Polish border. She was only seven years old when she made this journey. Aunt Lena lived in Queens with her husband, Julius, a tailor, who developed a chronic kidney condition and died young. Lena and Julius had two children, Irene and Alvin. After Julius died, Lena survived by taking on babysitting work for the women who lived in the big houses that surrounded her apartment in Queens.

Aunt Lena had long been my favorite woman of her generation. After Bessie died—the one who saw something in me beyond the skinny, hyper-anxious kid I was back then—Lena became my surrogate grandmother. My family looked forward to her visits each winter.

She stayed in our guest room, looked after our young daughters, prepared delicious soups, stewed chickens, baked kugels and challahs, all ready and waiting on the table when we finally dragged ourselves home at the end of each workday. These annual visits—which began when she was seventy-one and I was thirty-two—went on for many years. She stopped for a year or two, pleading fatigue, but when Aunt Lena was eighty-seven, I convinced her to come again. For once she looked her age; she was shuffling around, unsteady on her feet. Shortly after she arrived I took her to dinner with all her San Antonio family. She hated to see me pay good money for overpriced restaurant food and ordered only a salad. As we headed back to the car, her arm in mine until the last instant, she stumbled in a pothole and fell—just out of my grasp—cracking ribs and puncturing a lung.

She needed a week in the intensive care unit and many more of rest before she was strong enough to return to New York. Every day I examined her as I made my rounds, listening to her heart, checking her lungs for fluid, feeling her liver and spleen for pain, squeezing her calf muscles in search of clots.

"You got to see all my furniture," she told me. But she wasn't embarrassed. To have her great nephew, Bessie's grandson, minister to her needs was an honor for her.

I suspected that her gait change, slight tremor, and frozen facial features were caused by Parkinson's disease, and I started her on medications to treat this condition. I also discontinued a myriad of drugs prescribed by an array of medical and paramedical "professionals" whose only redeeming quality, as far as I could tell, was that they all were within walking distance of her apartment in Queens. Finally, she was ready to go back home.

"I think this will be the last visit for me," she said. "Another *alter kaker* with problems, you don't need. It used to be I could cook for you, bake *rugelach*, be of some use. Now I'm too much trouble."

"Aunt Lena," I said, "we don't have you visit every year just so you can cook for us! The kids love you. You're the only 'grandma' I've got left."

She thought for a moment. "For Bessie, if I can, I will be back."

But she didn't return that next year. Her daughter, Irene, called me. "You wouldn't recognize her. She's an old woman now. Won't eat. Can't sleep. Sits and stares. She can't visit you anymore." As soon as I could, I took some time off and flew to New York.

Her appearance frightened me. Her clothes hung on her. Her facial expression was devoid of emotion. Her hair was in disarray. A diminutive woman at her best, she was shrinking. I bent over to hug her.

"I'm ashamed you should see me like this," she said. "I knew you were coming, and I couldn't find the strength to cook, not even a chicken."

I started rummaging through her hall closet. "Aunt Lena," I said, "I didn't come here to eat. Where's your coat? Let's go for a walk in the park like we always do."

"I don't go there," she said. "I don't want for the neighbors to see me like this." But she reached into the closet and with great effort took out her old brown overcoat.

"Well, you're going outside with me now." I locked her arm in mine.

We walked slowly because she was shuffling badly again. I babbled about how the neighborhood always looks the same—"ageless," I said—expecting her to make a crack about the "aging" residents. But she said nothing, just shook her head. We sat on a park bench together in the late winter chill, my arm around her.

When we got back to her apartment, I asked to see her medications. She was no longer taking what I had prescribed and was back on a lot of other pills I didn't think she needed.

"Aunt Lena," I said, "I'm not giving up on you! You need a good doctor. And a psychiatrist. You're depressed."

"I don't need no psychiatrist! Irene sees enough psychiatrists for both of us! She's still a nervous wreck and smokes like a chimney!"

"We're not talking about Irene!" I was yelling now and I tried to calm down. "I'm going to see that you get help!"

"You need a sick, old woman like a *loch in kop*—a hole in the head!" she said.

When I walked into her bathroom and flushed all those pills down the toilet—pain pills, sleeping pills, bladder drugs, a dizzying accumulation of over-the-counter herbal remedies—she knew I meant business. This was a magnitude of waste she had never witnessed.

I started making phone calls and was soon armed with the names of a few physicians whom I contacted and screened. With Irene's help, we set up visits with a geriatrician, a neurologist, and a psychiatrist, and arranged transportation. I made sure I was kept apprised of Aunt Lena's progress. Occasionally, I put in my two cents' worth regarding some drug combination or other, and sent samples from my office whenever I had them—"to make up for all the pills I flushed down the toilet."

Within six months my aunt was her old self again.

She volunteered at a local hospital, wheeling patients to the dining room, where it was her mission to feed the ones who were poor eaters or unable to feed themselves. At this she was zealous. She joined the Ladies' Auxiliary of a synagogue near her home. She attended luncheons, sat in on lectures and discussion groups. She kept a strictly kosher kitchen again.

The next winter, when she was almost eighty-nine, I invited her to visit San Antonio once again. She was involved with the Auxiliary Bazaar at the time I suggested but promised to come soon. She told me how much she was enjoying her life now: "All the years I babysat for those women who would go to the luncheons, to hear the speakers. What I missed! Now it is my time to go."

For her birthday I sent her roses. She called to thank me but chastised me at the same time. "Don't send me any more birthday presents! I've had enough birthdays!"

"Only if you promise to come next year," I said.

"If I should be lucky to live so long, I'll come."

"Good. I need you." At the time I didn't know just how much.

One Friday morning—in my eighteenth year of practice—I received a call from a patient, a woman I had cared for over many years. Her thirty-year-old son, Jason, was ill and she asked me to work him in.

"Please, Doctor Winakur . . . I'm worried about him and he doesn't have a regular doctor anymore. Please see him today!"

Of course, I saw Jason. He was a diabetic, but his symptoms that day were vague, a little nausea and stomach upset. His physical examination was normal and none of his laboratory studies were out of line.

"Jason," I said, "I think perhaps you have a viral infection, but I certainly see nothing seriously wrong. Stay on liquids and take some Tylenol over the weekend and I'll see you Monday. If you get worse in any way, come into the emergency room and they'll call me."

"Okay, Doctor. Thanks for seeing me today. I know my mom appreciates it, too."

On Monday morning as I was dressing for work, his mother called me. Jason had just been found dead by his young wife. "My God. I am so sorry, so very sorry . . ." That was all I could think to say.

I rushed over to my office. Blood pulsed in my ears; bile refluxed in my throat. I reviewed my notes, the lab work. Nothing. There was an autopsy. Still nothing. To this day I don't know what happened to Jason. I went to his funeral mass, cried with his mother, hugged his wife, told them again how sorry I was.

But I stopped eating. I couldn't sleep. I quickly lost twenty pounds. I could find no joy in anything, not even my children. I never missed a day of work, but I found myself obsessing over each and every patient, third- and fourth-guessing myself. At home, late at night, I sat up in the living room to deal with my grief alone. My wife finally had enough. "You've got to snap out of this" she said. "Look what you're doing to us!" I made an appointment to see a psychiatrist.

Then a letter came from a local lawyer, the one whose face peers down from billboards and graces the back cover of the phone book, below the words in bold red type: *HAVE YOU OR A LOVED ONE BEEN WRONGFULLY INJURED?* He requested Jason's records. It was almost a relief—now I would be punished for what I had done. Even if I didn't know what mistake I had made, surely there was something. I would be exposed as the fraud I must be.

But after I sent off the records, I never heard another word about it. Apparently the lawyer and his team of hired experts couldn't find a reason to sue me. But I couldn't forgive myself. What was I—what kind of a doctor—if something like this could happen to one of my patients? Jason's mother continued to come to me and we mourned anew at every visit. But I was still losing weight. I still couldn't sleep.

Months passed and it was time for Aunt Lena to visit again. At the age of ninety she made the trip alone and I was at the airline gate with a wheelchair to greet her.

Lena took one look at me.

"What's the matter, are you sick? You're working too hard! Doctors in New York don't work so hard!"

I tried to change the subject. "You look terrific!" I said. "So much better than last time."

"That was a woman you brought back from the dead," she said, kissing me hard on both cheeks. "Don't tell me how good I look—I don't need a *keynahore*—no evil eye. But you—you're so thin!"

"Give me a break, Aunt Lena," I said. "I've been on a diet—trying to lose a few pounds, bring my cholesterol down . . . kind of like a vegetarian . . ."

"I make a delicious vegetarian chopped liver," she said, "out of green beans. You won't be able to tell the difference."

And then, "Why the wheelchair?" she asked.

"I brought the chair up here in case you were too tired or couldn't walk," I said. "I guess you don't need it, do you?"

"The stewardess also asked if I needed a wheelchair. I said, 'Why would I need a wheelchair when I have two legs that can walk still?' "

I offered her my arm and took her carry-on—after a brief skirmish over it—and we headed to the baggage area. I filled her in on the family news: my two daughters on the brink of college, a progress report on my aging parents. "My father can't wait to see you," I said.

"He's such a sweet man," Lena said. "Of all my nieces, Frances married the best one." And then, "*Oy vey,* my Irene. I can't believe I have a seventy-year-old daughter who isn't yet married." By then we had reached the baggage claim; I didn't have the energy to get into a discussion about Irene just yet.

"Point out your bags to me, Aunt Lena. How many are there?"

"Just one. A small one," she said. "How much clothes can a person use in two weeks? I'm not Irene—she comes for two weeks with five bags! There it is." That one she insisted on carrying herself.

I saw the psychiatrist weekly for about six months, started medication, talked endlessly about my mother and father and my childhood in their home, relived my great sadness over the loss of Grandma Bessie, defended the solidity of my marriage and the satisfaction—despite the stress—I got from practicing medicine.

"I don't know why I can't get past this thing," I said to him almost every visit.

One day, at the end of a session, he leaned toward me.

"I want to tell you one of the secrets of life," he said quietly.

I sat up in my chair. My senses were primed. I had been waiting for guidance, for wisdom. At last.

"In this life," he said, "you cannot be responsible for anyone's happiness but your own."

I sat there for a moment. I thought long and hard on his words. It made so much sense. I felt something shift deep inside me.

"Okay," I said. "Yes." I stood and shook his hand. He said he would see me the following week as usual.

By the time I reached my car in the parking lot, I couldn't remember what he had told me.

"I'm running behind," I said to Aunt Lena when she picked up the phone. "Don't wait dinner for me."

"We'll wait," she said. "It's *Shabbes*."

After eight that night, as the garage door groaned down, I walked into the kitchen to a joyful scene. A silver-haired old woman was ladling matzo ball soup into bowls. My grandmother's brass candlesticks flickered on the table. The smell of a roasting chicken came from the oven. A braided challah poked out from under a white linen napkin, awaiting the blessing.

"Wash up your hands and sit down. You must be starving," Aunt Lena said.

She watched me eat. She looked ready to jump up at any moment and *klop* me on the shoulder to force a swallow. I ate until I felt stuffed but left most of the food on my plate.

I had another sleepless night and was sitting up in the living room when Lena padded in on slippered feet so quietly that I didn't realize she was standing beside me. She set a tray down with a chicken sandwich, tea, and *rugelach*.

"Thanks, Aunt Lena. I'll do the best I can, but I'm really too tired to eat anything right now."

"Never mind. You need your strength. You work so hard. *Ess!*"

She sat next to me and watched as I began to eat. She moved her own jaw to get mine to chew. She didn't say anything until the food was gone. "It's good," I said.

"Aunt Lena, I know I haven't been very good company this visit." I took her knotted hand in mine. Her skin was warm and still so soft.

"You're so sad . . . so depressed! What's wrong?" she asked, her other hand on my chin, swiveling my head so she could peer into my eyes.

"Oh, I've just been working too hard. You know, I'm not getting any younger . . . like you."

"And you lost a lot of weight. Too much. How can you eat just vegetables, not even a chicken once in a while?" she said. "You're going to make yourself sick!"

"I wish I had your strength," I said. "I think your generation was the last of the *shtarkers,* the strong ones."

"Never mind. Bessie and me struggled to make a better life for our children, so they wouldn't have to struggle so much. And you are doing the same. Look how hard you work, all the hours, all the calls, day and night. This is easy? For this you don't need to be a *shtarker?*"

"Yes, you do, Aunt Lena," I said. I took a deep breath, ready to put into words what I never thought I could admit to anyone. "I don't think I was ever cut out for this doctoring life."

"How can you say this?" She took my face back into her hands. "You've been a doctor for so many years! You have a big practice, you help so many people . . ."

I didn't want to say any more, but it just came.

"I lost a patient recently. A young man. I don't know what happened to him but I just can't seem to get over it . . ."

"He was your patient for a long time?" she asked.

"No, I only saw him once." It all started coming back; I began to take slow, deep breaths.

"*Bashert,*" she said to me.

"What does that mean?"

"*Bashert.* Meant to be. Fated."

"No, I can't believe that."

"Why? You are perfect?" she said, an edge to her voice. "All doctors are perfect? Every doctor has his own graveyard. Look at my Julius, at your grandmother. Maybe there was something more to be done, maybe not. The doctors did the best they could and I don't think they lost sleep over it, neither. If there is only one patient in your graveyard after all these years, it proves you are a very good doctor. You want to eat up your insides because you're not perfect? What about your wife and children who love you and need you? What about all of your other patients who depend on you? No, you must be strong and go on. You *are* strong!"

"I've been trying, but . . ."

" 'But' nothing! You know that we believe that there is a record, a balance sheet, on all of us. Every year Jews pray that God should recognize our good deeds, forgive our bad ones. Look at your wonderful record! You are a good person and a fine doctor! Grandma Bessie would be proud of you. I wish she were here in my place to see you."

I hugged her and was hugged in return. A strong hug, like between two women.

My aunt Lena saved me that night. Her forthright words, her wisdom, hard-earned over a long and difficult life, helped me put my problems and my uncertainties into perspective. This is what families are for. This is why the elderly among us have traditionally held such an esteemed position in societal hierarchies. I fear that this is changing now in America.

Sadly today—for all of us but especially for our elderly—we live in a vain, youth-worshipping society, a society that, in every possible way, tells us that we must look young in order to feel young in order to be valued. The faces and bodies in magazine ads for incontinence products or the TV commercials for erectile dysfunction drugs do not in any way represent a fair cross section of my geriatric practice. The American Association of Retired People (AARP), one of the strongest lobbying and image-making groups in the nation, always has a movie star or celebrity on the cover of its glossy magazine—often someone who has been "made over" almost to the point of being unrecognizable.

Many of my patients—the old, the old old, and even the oldest old—are steadfast and stoic. They are the bedrock of their families. They bring loved ones into their homes and even take out second mortgages to support their children and their grandchildren. Sixty-two percent of multi-generational households—a growing phenomenon in America today—are led by the grandparents. My father picked my daughters up from elementary school every day, brought them to his house, fixed them snacks, taught them how to draw, read to them. My wife and I were able to carry on, knowing that our children were cared for and well loved in our absence.

My patients volunteer as "Bluebirds" in my hospital. Every day of the week I see folks like my patient, Mr. Burns—just a month or so after his own heart bypass surgery—wheeling other patients with acute illnesses to X-ray, to therapy. My hospital couldn't function without people like him.

Seniors support art and cultural events with their time and money. They work in the soup kitchens feeding the poor and hungry. They tutor youngsters in their schoolwork. I know a man, near ninety now, who has single-handedly organized adult education classes that have enlightened a generation of retired folks. Many elders are artists, painters, and writers, leading creative and productive lives that should inspire us all.

My aunt Lena lived to be one hundred and two years old. Her body gave out but her mind never did. She spent a couple of years in an assisted living facility and then in a nursing home not far from her apartment in Queens. Her daughter, Irene, now in her eighties, was her tireless advocate. Lena's son commuted to New York regularly to see her, but it was Irene—this daughter who bore the brunt of her mother's frustration and basked in her fierce love—who was steadfast and vigilant in the face of less-than-empathic caregivers and hard-nosed administrators.

When Lena's time came, neither Irene nor Alvin wanted to let go. There were many trips to the hospital and back to the nursing home until finally there was nothing more to do. I hope I was able to help them from afar through those times. I tried.

Aunt Lena has been gone a number of years now. I think about her often. Sometimes, when life is difficult, when I am haunted late at night by events I wish I could change but cannot, I dream about her. I am on foot in a big city—familiar yet not my own. I come to a thoroughfare where cars and taxis, buses and trucks, whiz by. On the other side is a little village, houses with white fences, small shops, chickens pecking in the yards, cows grazing contentedly in the fields. My heart races and I feel the sweat under my shirt. I sense I am going home, that somehow I must try to make it back. And then I am scampering in the traffic, horns blaring around me, the sound of squealing brakes and throbbing engines above me, sirens screaming from all directions. Spinning spotlights blind me as I bob and weave in this river of angry vehicles. I am paralyzed, stare up into tire treads bearing down, deep as graves. When there is nothing else to do, nowhere else to turn, I give myself over to fate—and feel my hand grasped by a soft gnarled one. Startled, I am floating behind a stooped, white-haired old woman—as in a painting by Chagall—as she leads me, so slowly, shuffling across the highway to the other side.

SIX

I didn't start out to be a geriatrician. I became one because my patients and I have grown old together. As a young internist, I began seeing many people in their fifties and sixties. Like my father thirty years ago, these folks needed management of their hypertension, their blood sugar and cholesterol levels. They needed their annual checkups, their mammograms and Pap smears, their prostate examinations, their routine colon cancer screens.

Over the years I dealt with each problem as it arose, did my best to counsel, to educate. Of course, I lost patients along the way, but now, three decades later, I am almost sixty and most of the people in my practice are in their seventies and eighties, many in their nineties. To keep up with them, with the knowledge base necessary to deal with the problems arising in their old, old years and beyond—their physical obsolescence, their dementias, their requirements for long-term care, their families' need for guidance as the end of life approaches—I continued to study the latest developments in clinical geriatrics, sat for my "added qualifications in geriatrics" board examination, and did it again ten years later when the initial certification expired. Likewise, I have twice fulfilled the requirements to become a long-term-care medical director. All this—a lifetime of ongoing learning and experience—and still I often feel inadequate in the face of the tasks that confront me day in and day out, with my patients and my own father.

The practice of geriatric medicine differs from other medical specialties, even internal medicine and family practice, which share overlapping patient populations. Geriatrics is not just about treating and triumphing over disease. There is no triumph over aging, after all.

A geriatrician and the editor of the journal *Geriatrics*, Dr. Fred Sherman, reflects on the art of observing his elderly patients: "Can a woman get out of a chair without pushing off with her hands? That means she can still use the toilet. Can a man put on his socks? If not, he will soon need someone to dress and bathe him." Geriatrics is very much about trying to maintain the functional status of our patients, doing the best we can to keep them independent, safe, and happy. And in order to manage this, our loved ones—my patients—must be, at the most basic level, able to get in and out of bed, feed and groom themselves, as well as shop, cook, handle their financial affairs, and take their medications correctly. If at all possible, I want to help them postpone their frailty, avoid falls, and maintain their social connections to family and friends.

Geriatricians are protective of their patients. We shield them from the hucksters of the "anti-aging" and pharmaceutical industries, even from our own colleagues who, at times, are unrealistic about how easy it will be to put in that new knee or bypass that blocked artery.

Many years ago, when my father first came to San Antonio, he developed a hernia. My friend, a general surgeon, a man I trust and admire, repaired it. Now my father has developed another hernia. His surgeon feels that it ought to be fixed. We both worry that it might become trapped in the groin area; if it does, it could kill my father. But I also worry—geriatricians worry—about the delirium that will develop in-hospital, the depression that might follow prolonged recuperation, the deconditioning that occurs with enforced bed rest, the infection that might flare in the post-op period.

"Is your hernia bothering you," I ask my father regularly.

"What are you talking about?" he says.

"That lump you have in your groin, Dad. Does it hurt?"

He feels around inside his pajamas. "I don't even know it's there," he says.

I figure my father will likely die with his hernia, not from it. And I am willing to accept the consequences if I am wrong.

We geriatricians are in for the long haul with our patients. Of course, we want to stem the tide of disease if we can. But we also know that one day we won't be able to hold back that tide. We want to be there at those most trying times, marshalling resources, motivating the other members of the geriatric team, educating and preparing the family.

Perhaps most of all, geriatricians, like most good primary care doctors, understand the difference between pain and suffering.

Suffering is not confined to physical symptoms and is not even necessarily related to the disease process itself but often to the treatment of the disease, which, in this time of toxic chemotherapy regimens and immune system assaults, can often be worse than the original illness itself. Unless a patient is asked by her physician—a process that takes time, takes probing—to talk about the source and nature of her suffering, *not pain but suffering*, the doctor may never really sound the depths of the problem and never help the patient.

My medical training did not directly address the issue of suffering. Even today this subject is too often ignored in medical schools. Laypersons, Dr. Eric Cassel notes, are shocked to discover this. As he observes:

> *The relief of suffering, it would appear, is considered one of the primary ends of medicine by patients and laypersons, but not by the medical profession. As in the care of the dying, patients . . . do not make a distinction between physical and non-physical sources of suffering in the same way that doctors do.*

Until doctors understand our patients as *persons*—their personality, character, fears, cultural background, spiritual life, and hopes for the future—we can never appreciate the reasons for or the depths of their suffering. This knowledge of another person takes time, and this is hard to come by in our age when technology is replacing personal relationships, when doctor-patient encounters get squeezed into shorter and shorter time frames.

It takes a special commitment—"a calling" was the term once used—to choose a career in geriatrics. Medical students start out full of idealism, but as their years of training grind on, many of them undergo a transformation. I witness this change each spring when I help teach the Humanities and Ethics module for the fourth-year students. I walk in to greet my new small group. They have been through the wringer, have figured out for themselves that there is often a fine line between what is Hippocratic and what is hypocrisy. Many are jaded and cynical now. Most of them are deeply in debt after college and medical school.

They are waiting for Match Day when fourth-year medical students in America learn where they will be going for residency training. I look around the room; I sense many of them would rather not be here. It's spring; their formal course work is almost complete. They are ready to get on with their lives, impatient with "ethics."

"So, tell me what you each hope to be doing come July," I say.

"Radiology," says a woman in the front row. She has a big smile, bright teeth.

"Orthopedics," a young man in tennis shorts chimes in, his muscled well-tanned legs splayed out.

"Dermatology," says another young woman sitting right in front of me. She is beautiful, blond. There is not a blemish on her face.

"Cardiology," says another. She is tapping on her BlackBerry.

"And what about you?" I ask, pointing to a student in the back of the room. She has shy brown eyes, dark bangs covering her forehead. "Pediatrics," she says.

"Great!" I say.

It goes on like this for a while. I identify two future ophthalmologists, a plastic surgeon, a gastroenterologist, two heart surgeons, and a gene researcher.

When I first became a doctor, I was proficient in a few diagnostic procedures that I used only when I needed to answer a specific question or save a life. I could do a spinal tap if I feared my patient might have meningitis, could glide a needle into the chest or abdominal cavity to aid in the diagnosis of an infection or malignancy. I learned how to intubate a patient about to stop breathing, finesse a length of plastic tubing into someone's veins to give fluid or blood or monitor pressures. I could snake a rubber catheter into a distended bladder to relieve a urinary obstruction or down a gullet to provide temporary sustenance.

I always considered that my ability to perform these few procedures was a peripheral activity, secondary to my real role as a diagnostician, an expert on therapeutics, a patient advocate, and a family resource in troubled times.

Today medicine is all about procedures. Our ability to invade the body, collect specimens, and image the deepest organs has advanced to such a degree that it is impossible to practice state-of-the-art medicine without using these modern techniques. I depend on the information my cardiologist provides after he has skillfully negotiated a catheter through my patient's arteries and injected dye into her coronaries at the base of her aorta. Are her chest pains a sign that these vessels are about to close? Does she need bypass surgery tonight? Can we get by with a tiny stent that the cardiologist might guide into place now to relieve her pain and maybe even save her life?

My gastroenterologist colleague maneuvers his scope through the pink tunnel of colon, snipping out polyps and even small cancers that much earlier in my career required the services of a general surgeon and all the morbidity and mortality that general anesthesia and major abdominal surgery entails.

Every day as I practice medicine now, my patients benefit from the technological advances I have witnessed: stereotactic biopsies of tiny abnormalities on mammograms frequently save much larger and more disfiguring procedures; prostatic ultrasound and biopsies diagnose cancer in this organ at the earliest stages; percutaneous injection of special cements repair osteoporotic spine and pelvic fractures and relieve terrible pain that doctors found almost impossible to assuage in past years.

Thus, the trend today is toward even more specialization: "Hospitalists" manage acutely ill patients while "intensivists" monitor their stays in ICUs; "proceduralists" are called upon to perform this or that invasive study but otherwise have no role in ongoing patient care. These trends tend to crowd out the primary care doctor, the one who knows the patient and her family and has her trust. Indeed, many insurance companies now insist that once a patient requires hospital admission, the primary doctor must relinquish total care of her patient to one or more of these specialists.

I am not convinced that this is entirely a positive trend. I worry that my patients may be subjected to procedures that are ill-advised, ones they do not need or even want, in the rush to do "everything that is possible." I worry about gaps in care—the transitions between my office and the hospital, skilled units, and nursing homes—that occur because there are "too many cooks in the kitchen." I worry that sometimes a procedure is performed just because someone is available to perform it—and the insurance company will pay for it. I cannot but ask: Who is now "on call" as patient advocate in this brave new world of high-tech medicine?

The acquisition of procedural skills without reasoned, practiced judgment is a bit like sitting a Boy Scout behind the console of an aircraft carrier and saying, "Have at it, son." Procedural medicine without trained and knowledgeable operators—those who order the tests and interpret the results—is dangerous. It exposes patients to risks for no real benefit and, often, produces insignificant results or "red herrings"—which only necessitate additional testing and thus even more risk.

So I am troubled by the brochures I receive regularly in the mail: *Are you working harder and earning less?* the flyer asks. *Procedures increase your profits without any extensive training!* For a few hundred dollars and a weekend of my time I can learn one of these skills: laser aesthetics, nasopharyngoscopy, infrared coagulation of hemorrhoids, radiofrequency electrosurgery, sclerotherapy, and "no-scalpel" vasectomy.

The promotions promise that I will have a better relationship with my patients because I can treat their everyday problems myself and avoid sending them to high-cost specialists. *This course will pay for itself in the next few weeks,* the brochure says. It says nothing about who—if anyone—really needs many of these procedures.

Tremendous income disparities exist today between medical specialties. These differences have little to do with the number of years a practitioner has trained, his experience and dedication to his patients, or his work ethic or lack of it. These disparities exist only because insurance companies, lobbying groups, and government programs—Medicare the most egregious of these—have decided that "procedures" are more valuable than "cognitive" services: thinking, reasoning, examining and interpretation skills. These groups have decreed that technological gimmicks—the latest and greatest devices and procedures—deserve higher reimbursements.

This has led to an oversupply of specialists and a dearth of primary care doctors like me. Twenty-one percent of physicians once certified by the internal medicine (IM) board in the 1990s have left the field, as compared to only 5 percent of subspecialists. In 1998, 54 percent of third-year IM residents planned a career in general internal medicine; in 2003 this percentage fell by one half. Any policymaker who wants to seriously address the crisis in primary care that already exists in America—especially in geriatrics—and which is predicted to worsen in the decades to come, should consider the discrepancies in Medicare reimbursement. Here is an example:

An eighty-year-old woman calls my office one morning and tells my secretary that she has had some kind of a "spell." We know her well, recognize that she has diabetes and high blood pressure, takes a long list of medications, and is at risk for something serious. She comes to see me that day. We do not send her into the din of the emergency room or admit her directly into the hospital for a battery of tests. I talk to her, pin down the circumstances of her "spell"—how it came on, what the exact symptoms were that she associates with the episode. Was there chest pain, slurred speech, weakness, loss of consciousness, vertigo, nausea? I review her past medical history—has something like this occurred before? I look at her medications—the actual bottles she has been asked to bring in with her. We evaluate each one to make sure she is taking it as prescribed.

I examine her completely, head to toe. I narrow down the list of possibilities. A few simple tests done in my office and which I can have completed in minutes help me: a blood count, an EKG, a blood sugar and serum potassium level. I make a judgment that she needs further evaluation but that she is stable for now and can be set up for one or two studies as an outpatient: perhaps a sound-wave test of her carotid arteries to look for blockages, a further inner-ear evaluation. Maybe I think I can get by with a minor adjustment in her blood pressure medications or the addition of a small dose of aspirin to her regimen for the time being. Or maybe not. Maybe I decide she must go into the hospital now, today, for observation and more extensive testing.

I make a very important decision at this moment, but it is one I am well trained and experienced to make. It is still fraught with uncertainty and I am only too well aware of the potential consequences if I am wrong.

My patient trusts me because we know each other. Maybe I took care of her husband for years before he passed away. Perhaps her adult children are my patients. I discuss with her what my best guess is as to the cause of her "spell," how I'd like to proceed; what she should be on the lookout for in the way of additional symptoms should I send her home; why—should I decide this—she must go into the hospital today; what tests I intend to order and the reason for them.

She may refuse to take my advice. She may be afraid of going into the hospital. She may not want "a lot of tests run." We talk and talk. Nothing is written in stone. We can go about the evaluation in a different manner, another sequence. We can watch and wait. I will be available. I will see her in a week if not sooner. My nurse will call her tomorrow and check in. If I am away for some reason, one of my associates will have her chart with my thoughts and plan recorded in it and will take over for me.

Should I send her home, that is the end of my "billable encounter"—to use the terminology of the insurance industry. But it is not the end of my involvement in her care as a result of that office visit. There will be lab and X-ray results to review, phone calls to patient and family and consultants, follow-up letters drafted and sent. And nowadays there are faxes and e-mails to deal with. All of this additional effort in coordination—and worry—is time-consuming and ongoing. To make matters worse, a recent study has shown that more than twenty-two percent of the time devoted to patient care coordination by geriatricians in an ambulatory care practice is unreimbursed by Medicare and other third parties. I wonder how my local grocer would feel if he had to give away every fifth shopping bag full of his wares to each customer. How long would he remain in business?

Still, day in and day out, this is how I practice medicine, how I approach each and every patient. There is nothing remarkable or startling about it. Nothing high-tech. Most of my primary care colleagues practice medicine in some similar fashion. And because we do, the overall cost of health care is significantly lower than for patients seen only by specialists.

But why not choose a simpler doctoring life: remove the mole, read the CT scan, do the procedure, go home for a quiet night with the family and forget about the patient?

The "comprehensive follow-up visit" (to use Medicare's definition) of the doctor-patient encounter I have just described takes me anywhere from thirty to sixty minutes. There are only so many hours in the day that I can keep my office open, that I have the energy to work.

For my efforts, Medicare mandates a fixed payment to me of x dollars, with yearly adjustments; some years, negative adjustments occur, and these days cuts in physician reimbursements are perpetually threatened. This sum of x dollars was first calculated by Medicare wonks and actuaries in 1992, based on something called the "resource-based relative-value scale" (RVU). This has been a sore point with primary doctors ever since and it has turned out that the main driver for RVU increases has been for procedures, not the kind of "cognitive" services that I provide. Primary care doctors—especially those in the field of geriatric long-term care—have been and remain very disappointed in Medicare for putting this RVU system into place, as it was "based on assumptions reflecting no clear understanding of (long-term care) and the work it involved." It is no secret to any privately practicing doctor today—no matter what their specialty—that "current reimbursement incentives substantially favor procedures and technical interventions and offer financial advantages for expensive care . . ."

Here are some examples that only begin to scratch the surface of our perverse system: If I were in an ER and had just sutured a one-inch laceration—a technical act that takes minutes—I would get about the same amount I received for the patient visit I described, or "x" dollars for my efforts. If I had become a gastroenterologist, I could pass a scope through a colon and get $3x$. Remove a mole and collect almost $3x$. Interpret an echocardiogram (performed remotely by a technician)—as cardiologists do—and get $3x$. Or do a stress test—another technician-performed procedure—and collect $6x$ from Medicare. Had I become a radiologist, I could sit in a darkened room and read MRI scans—and collect almost $9x$ per study.

Believe it or not, my ear, nose, and throat colleague is reimbursed almost as much by Medicare to clean the wax out of my elderly patient's ear during an office visit as I receive for the above encounter I described.

To add insult to injury, the RVU system is codified and perpetuated by none other than the American Medical Association (AMA) through their secretive and subspecialist-stacked "Resource-based Relative Value Scale Update Committee (RUC)." Twenty-three of the thirty members are appointed by medical specialty societies, and the meetings are closed and proprietary. "Seventeen of the permanent seats on the RUC are assigned to . . . specialty societies . . . that account for a very small portion of all professional Medicare billing, such as neurosurgery, plastic surgery, pathology, and otolaryngology." And over 90 percent of this committee's recommendations are enacted by Medicare. Traditionally, primary care doctors have been too busy seeing patients, too busy scrambling to keep their doors open to lobby effectively in the corridors of power. So perhaps we are partly to blame. Our interests have not been well served by our specialty colleagues who live by our referrals.

There are those who will accuse me of sour grapes. To them I will answer that I chose my medical path many years ago and I am satisfied with my lot. I would make the same choice today.

In the 2007–08 academic year, students applied to medical school in unprecedented numbers, continuing to reverse a downward trend that occurred in the years 1998–2002. These students—most of whom are truly interested in serving their fellow human beings—are responding to our nation's growing awareness of the impending critical doctor shortage. If America can rebuild its base of primary care physicians, we can begin to cut the cost of health care and improve patient satisfaction with that care.

If policy-makers fix these egregious reimbursement disparities, young doctors will once again feel that they can spend their lives doing face-to-face primary care medicine. They want to do it; they are dis-heartened that they cannot do it and pay back their loans (currently averaging over \$100,000 from public medical schools and \$135,000 from private ones), open an office, pay their overhead expense (50–60 percent today in primary care) and their yearly malpractice premiums (for me, now equal to one month's take-home pay).

Unfortunately, I see little effort on the part of those in power to correct these disparities. It will take a grass-roots movement by patients—not doctors—if the status quo is to change. That may well happen as more and more of our citizens—especially our elderly—are unable to find a competent doctor to care for them. Recent calls by medical organizations for "specialists" to become better versed in car-ing for the geriatric patient's general medical needs sound like wishful thinking to me.

At a time in our nation's history when a baby boomer turns sixty every eight seconds, when only about three hundred doctors begin a career in geriatric medicine each year (fewer than those retiring), and when the current deficit of doctors trained to care for the oldest among us will rise from fourteen thousand to thirty-four thousand by 2030, it is time for public policy to catch up to this reality: In our "Golden Years" who will *minister* to us and not just *do things* to us?

In the face of all of this, each spring I give my fourth-year medical students an ethics pep talk, a real-world primer on the importance of the subject.

I ask them to pause for just a moment, to think back over their last four years. I want them to remember the sharp smell of the anatomy lab, the first time they drew back the sheets on their cadavers, the pages of diagrams and drawings they panicked to memorize—all those metabolic pathways, those chemical structures morphing into yet oth-ers along with those tricky enzymes doing this and that to carbon and oxygen, nitrogen and hydrogen atoms. It was an almost impossible task, yet somehow they did it, mastered the stuff of medicine: the parts of the human body from the smallest organic molecule to the largest organ. They learned how it all works, how it all fits together, how it can fall apart in disease and human aging. They mastered all this so they might be able to help others. I want them to remember that this is why they came here.

They are on the brink of their careers, but now they are required to attend another humanities/ethics module where the talk is sometimes abstract, sometimes philosophical. Where we read and discuss short stories like Nathaniel Hawthorne's "The Birthmark" and Richard Selzer's "Brute"; poems like William Carlos Williams's "Complaint" and W. S. Merwin's "To the Surgeon Kevin Lin." They are impatient, ready to get on with their doctoring lives.

I assure them that when I was where they are today, in 1973, I might have felt the same way. There was no course like this one then, so I didn't have to bother myself about it at all. I located the canal of Schlemm, memorized where in the grand metabolic schema the action of ornithine transcarbamylase kicked in. I never heard the words "autonomy" or "beneficence," "nonmaleficence," or "social justice" uttered in the lecture halls of my medical school, the wards of the hospital where I did my residency.

I want to make it relevant for these doctors-soon-to-be. I tell them about my own practice, my own patients, the ethical problems I confront every day. Put yourself in my place, I say: What would you do?

Your eighty-four-year-old patient, whose wife died two years ago and who is now living alone, is hospitalized with a mild stroke. Two days after admission he becomes confused, but this clears up quickly. You are ready to discharge him but realize he is still weak and needs more rehab work with physical therapy. When you enter his room, he says, "Please, Doctor, just let me go home. Whatever I need to do to get back on my feet, I'll do. Just let me go home. Please."

You are caring for an elderly demented woman who resides in a nursing home after several strokes. At the time of her last stroke, her

daughter—who is her designated surrogate decision-maker—begged
you to place a feeding tube into her mother's stomach. It is now three
months later, your patient is no better, and the daughter is demanding
that you withdraw nutritional support.

The nursing home calls to notify you that one of your patients, a
ninety-two-year-old man with severe Alzheimer's, has just undergone
"free" eye screening by a local ophthalmologist, who has discovered a
cataract. Your patient's son, who lives 1,200 miles away and whom
you have met just once, has faxed in a signed surgical consent form
authorizing this doctor to proceed with an operation. You know that
your patient has not been able to read or concentrate on a television
show for the past five years because his dementia is too advanced. You
are being asked to clear your patient medically for this operation.

Your seventy-six-year-old patient with diabetes, hypertension,
and high cholesterol comes to you for a routine visit and says, "Doc-
tor, I'm really having a hard time paying for my medicines. Sometimes
it comes down to buying food or buying drugs. A friend told me that
I can get them a lot cheaper in Canada. What do you think?"

I see that their responses are tentative; they are uncertain. I tell
them not to worry, that they are way ahead of where I once was, that
the answers will come with time and experience. I let them know
how much I admire them, envy their fresh beginning at this most
critical time in the history of medical care in our nation, that I am
looking forward to hearing their voices speak out for the good of our
profession and the health care of our citizenry.

Finally, I assure them that if they will open their minds, free them
from certain dogmas of personal philosophy, if they develop a frame-
work based on the few basic ethical principles we will discuss over
and over, if they learn always to first identify with the patient amid
the blizzard of data and demands of families, if they realize that sometimes a colleague and often the system itself is ailing, if they remember that one day each one of them will be the patient, then I
guarantee they will be wiser, more compassionate physicians earlier

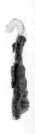

in their careers than I was. They will be able to reason through some tough problems and help each other and their patients make complex decisions. They will know more clearly what their role is, where it begins and ends. And finally—no small reward—they will sleep better at night.

They are listening to me now. I have their attention, for how long I don't know. But I must tell them this: You will never have all the answers, you will never be perfect, you will make mistakes. But you are not alone. Look around. These are your colleagues. Cherish them, talk to them, support them. One day you will need someone to help you.

SEVEN

When I look at my father—his twisted frame, his lined face, his wasted muscles—I see myself. Each time my father and I talk I am newly saddened when I confront the great swaths of memory now lost to him, even the ones we shared together and which, for the moment at least, are still so vivid in my own mind: the time we were lost in the fog off Thomas Point, the low monotonous drone from the lighthouse our only guide to safety; the peregrine falcon we saw hovering above the salt flats of Copano Bay, both of us mesmerized as it plunged earthward into a skein of blue-winged teal. When I can't remember a name or misplace my keys, my first thought is, *I am becoming my father.*

I have heard it said that our parents are our bulwarks against our own impending mortality, that as long as they are alive we have the illusion of believing we can live forever. They have been around our entire lives; they will always be around. What can possibly happen to that strong, loving man or woman, our father or our mother, our nurturer, our protector? And if nothing can happen to them, what could possibly happen to us?

My father and I have never been able to talk about death, let alone his death. It's as if to talk about the subject will hasten its arrival; to ignore it might stave it off. We can't talk about what kind of burial he would like, what he might want to do with his worldly possessions. I can't ask him about his fears or what brings him solace. I can only infer what he remembers as his happiest times, his greatest accomplishments, or his regrets.

Some of my patients talk incessantly about their illnesses. I try to reassure them that they are healthy for their age, make them a four-month appointment for a follow-up. They're back the next month and nothing has changed. Some are obsessed with death. They try to pin me down: "How long have I got, Doc, really? What do you think, five years, ten?"

"But there's nothing wrong with you," I say. "Okay, you're getting older, but so is everybody. The average life expectancy these days is almost eighty! You're not even close yet. Give yourself a break," I say.

"I've gotta make plans, Doc. You know."

Talking about and planning for death seems to be their way of dealing with it.

Unfortunately, neither of these approaches—denial or obsession—is a constructive way to handle this important issue. We need honest conversations among loving family members, a compassionate fearlessness in pursuing the truth about how a sick or aging parent wants the end to be, what he does and doesn't want in the way of medical intervention, how she wants to be remembered.

We must have these conversations before a crisis arises. By our reticence, because of our own fears about the end of life, we lose important opportunities to know each other better, to understand each other and our own selves, to learn how to pass a valuable life lesson along to our children.

Doctors deal with death all the time; it seems logical that their training should help them become more comfortable with it. This was not my experience as a medical student, and even today the subject is barely touched upon. Most doctors, like most people, are tongue-tied when the topic comes up, uncomfortable talking about death among themselves, let alone with their patients. So I begin a discussion with my students.

I hope I am getting through to these young men and women on the cusp of their professional lives, that they will be better able to deal with these issues of aging and death than I was at their age. But there is one more thing I want to know, and finally I get up the nerve to ask outright: "Is anyone in this room considering a career in geriatric medicine?"

In the back corner a young man tentatively raises his hand. His shoulders are slumped. I had watched him when he came into the room. He was carrying a paperback copy of Sinclair Lewis's *Arrowsmith*.

"Well," he says, "I'm doing an internal medicine residency and I'm thinking about geriatrics. But . . ."

"But what?"

"It's so sad," he says. "They all die . . ."

"It happens to the best of us," I say. Many of the students laugh. "But while 'they' are living, 'they'—and I will include myself in this category since I will be there soon—need good doctors like you. And there is no greater reward."

"Are you kidding?" he says. "Geriatrics is like the worst-paying specialty there is."

"You're right," I say. "But so am I."

I think to myself that if this one student out of twenty goes into geriatric medicine, my class will be above average in this regard. Poll them a year from now, during their residencies, and only two in a hundred will raise their hand.

Last week I admitted Mrs. Alder with a stroke. She has had a ten-year decline physically and mentally. Now she is on a respirator and tomorrow I will meet with her children about turning off the machine.

Yesterday Mr. Dillon came into the office black and blue from

having fallen in his kitchen, his third fall in the last six months. Fortunately, he has not broken anything—yet. His son lives in Maine
and insists that his father be allowed to live out the remainder of his
days at home even if there is no one around to look after him.

Last night my mother found my father in a heap, half-dressed,
inside the front door. Before he had gone to sleep, they'd watched
CNN together, extended footage of the Iraq war. "I've got to report
to my unit," my father said to her when she found him lying there.
"Nates and Sammy are waiting for me!"

"What's going to happen to him?" my mother says after I have
come over to their house and gotten my father back into his bed.
We are sitting in the kitchen. My mother has made me a cup of tea
I did not ask for.

"We have to talk about this, Mom. It's time."

"What do you mean?" she says.

"This isn't going to get any better."

"He still has good days . . ."

"He's going to fall and break his hip and that will be the beginning of the end for him. It could happen tomorrow. It could happen
tonight after I leave . . ."

"Your tea is getting cold," she says.

EIGHT

My mother calls me, distraught. "Your father refuses to take a shower. He hasn't had one all week. He won't even listen to Yolanda. What should I do?" After work, I head over there. My father is sitting on the couch, half asleep in his pajamas, unshaven. He looks like a homeless person. My mother has placed a towel underneath him in case he leaks urine. I sit down next to him. He smells fetid, overripe.

"Hello, Dad," I say.

He opens his eyes wide and looks into my face. "Is that you, Jerry-boy?"

"Who else?"

"What brings you around at this hour of the night?"

"I hear through the grapevine that you won't take a shower."

"Who told you that?" he says. "Did Mom tell you that?"

"It doesn't matter. Have you been refusing to take a shower?"

"I don't think so," he says.

"Well, to be perfectly honest, Dad, you smell like you haven't had a shower in a while."

He lifts his arm and sniffs his armpit.

"You're right," he says. "Maybe I need to take a shower."

"How 'bout I give you a hand?" I say.

"I'd appreciate that. You ought to come around more often, Jerry-boy."

"If you promise to take a shower whenever Yolanda asks you to, I'll come around more often."

"Who's Yolanda?" he says.

"Dad, you remember Yolanda. She's the really nice lady with the big smile who comes here almost every day to help you get dressed, who shaves you and helps bathe you. You like Yolanda, don't you?"

"Oh, yeah," he says. "Now I remember her. I like her fine."

"Well, Dad, you let her help bathe you and I'll come over more often. What do you say?"

"You got a deal, Jerry-boy."

Years before my father became overtly demented he started having problems emptying his bladder. After his visit to a urologist we had some tough decisions to make. He had cancer.

"Whatever you say, I'll do" was his initial reaction to the diagnosis.

I was surprised, because my father's usual response to my medical advice had been to question it.

"What do you know?" he'd say.

Once—I had been in practice for ten years at that point—I drove to his house late at night to bring him antibiotics for the bronchitis I'd suspected when my mother outlined his symptoms over the phone. I listened to his chest. He then proceeded to cough yellow sputum into his white handkerchief—which he presented to me, in case I might want to alter my diagnosis, perhaps to something more serious. I should have remembered that his distrust had everything to do with his own poor self-esteem and nothing to do with a lack of confidence in me, his son the doctor. But in those

years I still resented his failure to bounce back after he lost his business, and my responses to him were often harsh.

"*Now* you trust me?" I said. "Now that you've got prostate cancer?"

"You've had more practice," he said, his face reddening, an edge
to his voice.

"First of all, you don't have to undergo any treatment," I said,
trying to sound as professional as possible.

"So then I'll die," he said. "Is that what you want?"

"Of course not, Dad. It's just another option, that's all. Prostate
cancer is very slow growing. You're seventy-five years old with a bad
heart. You know I'll respect whatever choice you make."

"And the radiation?" He sat straight up in his usual seat at the old
black-and-white checkered kitchen table and looked across at me.

"I want you to understand all the potential side effects of the radiation," I said. "You might have trouble holding your urine. You will
probably have diarrhea until the rectum heals from the radiation, but
that will most likely get better over time."

"I'll have a mess on my hands," my mother said.

"That's what she worries about!" he said. As always, he looked at
me as if I should fix it for him, as if it were my fault.

"Mom, Dad . . ."

My mother started to cry, "See how mean he can be . . ."

Anger and sadness washed over me, something I have experienced
many, many times in my life as my parents' oldest son, the one to whom
they turned to smooth the rough edges of their often difficult marriage. Of course, this bickering between couples is not uncommon;
I've often witnessed it—been in the middle of it—in my office exam
rooms. It's always easier to deal with in someone else's parents.

"I'll come back later," I said as I rose to go. "Think about the options we discussed. We'll talk again. There's no rush. Remember,
prostate cancer grows slowly, and yours was picked up early."

I wanted to believe this, but when the urologist had called me with
the cancer diagnosis, I'd worried and, of course, visualized the worst:

malignant cells chewing spicules of bone as if they were after-dinner mints. I can't help it: Years of dealing with bad news and progressive diseases have me programmed to envision the worst, mourn at the time of diagnosis. This keeps me vigilant—and maybe I think I'll get the emotional part out of the way faster. But I never do.

My mother wept into the pink Kleenex she had extracted from the sleeve of her housecoat, where it was always at the ready. My father reached for the newspaper and picked up a pencil to work on the daily Jumble.

"Don't be a stranger," he said to me as I walked toward the front door.

"What do you want from him?" I heard my mother say. "He's a busy doctor!"

"I'll call tomorrow," I yelled from the stoop.

The night I had my first seizure, I was thirty-three years old, in practice for five years. All that day I'd felt achy, fighting off the flu, I'd thought. I had worked in the office, stopped at the hospital before coming home, and took some Tylenol before going to bed. My two young daughters came into my bedroom, rubbing their eyes, the oldest carrying *Cheaper by the Dozen*.

I read as long as I could, but as I was drifting off to sleep, book across my chest, I had a convulsion. The kids ran screaming for their mother, who was in the kitchen. "Daddy's choking! Daddy's choking!"

I remember waking up in the ambulance, asking the EMT what had happened, my mind running through a list of differential diagnoses, deciding I had either meningitis or a brain tumor. I hoped for the infection, figuring that with antibiotics I might survive intact.

My neurologist friend, Steve, met me in the ER, examined me thoroughly, noted my high fever, and finessed a needle through my back into my subdural space to collect a couple of vials of cerebrospinal fluid.

I lay on my side. He stood behind, watching the liquid drip into the plastic tube he was holding. "It's clear," he said. This was meant to reassure me, but I still worried about a brain tumor.

"That's great, Steve. Thanks for coming out tonight."

"You owe me one," he said.

After the spinal tap, I was lying on the stretcher in the hall outside the CT scanner—about to get the first pictures of the tumor I figured I must have—when they wheeled up Mr. Clark. Ten hours before I'd admitted him with a short-lived but worrisome episode of dizziness and confusion. I had ordered a CT scan of his brain.

"Dr. Winakur?" He turned on his side, pulling himself up using his right arm, the one that had been weak ten hours before. I was relieved; he was getting better. "Is that you, Doctor?"

"Don't worry, Mr. Clark," I said. "I'll be fine by tomorrow. Just have your tests done and I'll be around in the morning to go over everything with you and your wife." Steve was loading me up on Dilantin, an anticonvulsant; I knew I'd be in the office the next day, no matter what my scan showed.

"Are you sure?" Mr. Clark asked. "I want to get out of here tomorrow," he said. "Don't leave me hanging!"

"Don't worry about anything," I said as the tech came to roll me into the scanner. "Do him first," I said to the tech.

Steve had scheduled my brain wave test for 5 A.M. so it would be ready when he made rounds at seven, and so, if I hadn't seized again, I could get out in time to be in my office by nine.

He was smiling when he came in. "The CT was fine. Just a little right temporal lobe irritability on the brain wave."

"Where would that come from?" I asked, knowing full well the range of possibilities.

"Did you ever have a head injury—you know, maybe a car accident where you got banged around? Or an old sports injury, a concussion?"

"I don't know of anything," I said.

"Well, you know how these things are," he said. "Most of the time we never discover the original insult. Hey, it could have been a lot worse. You'll be fine."

"Sure," I said.

So Steve discharged me and I discharged Mr. Clark. "You'll be fine," I said to him—and I made it to the office only ten minutes late for my first patient, who was looking at her watch, shaking her head as I walked into the exam room.

A week after my conversation with my father about his newly diagnosed prostate cancer, I rang the doorbell of my parents' house.

"It's you again, so soon," my father said.

"Hush!" said my mother. Then to me, "You look tired. Did you eat?"

"I'm fine," I said. "Any decisions yet?"

"I thought you said there's no rush. What, am I dying here?" My father moved his hands toward me, palms up, over the kitchen table.

"I just wanted to know if you've been thinking about it."

"Whatever you say, I'll do," he said, his eyes avoiding mine.

"Think about it some more," I said.

Then for some reason, after all the years that had passed since my first seizure, I asked, "Did I ever fall down as a child? I mean, hit my head hard, maybe pass out for a few seconds? Anything like that?"

"You were a sickly child," said my mother. "You caught everything that came down the pike. But what kind of parents do you think we were . . . to let you fall and hit your head?" My father said nothing, sat with his hands clasped in front of him.

"Why do you ask?" said my mother. "What's wrong?"

"Nothing, nothing. . . . Just trying to fill in my past medical history, that's all."

"Are you sure?" my mother pressed. "There's nothing wrong?"

"Nothing." I got up to go.

"You need to lose some weight," my father said. He held his closed hand up to his mouth and blew into the hollow of his fist a few times, a nervous habit of his.

Physicians are always getting caught up in caring for friends or family members who are not really their patients in the traditional sense. The AMA calls these folks "non-patients" and sternly warns doctors against treating them. There are good reasons for this: Professional objectivity may be compromised and the physician's personal feelings may unduly influence his medical judgment. Physicians who put themselves in this situation may, in the words of the AMA . . .

> *fail to probe sensitive areas when taking the medical history or may fail to perform intimate parts of the physical examination. Concerns regarding patient autonomy and informed consent are also relevant when physicians attempt to treat members of their immediate family. Family members may be reluctant to state their preference for another physician or decline a recommendation for fear of offending the physician.*

All of these reasons are rational, reasonable, and, of course, ignored by most doctors. There is survey data demonstrating that treatment of "nonpatients" is widespread, with some studies reporting nearly 100 percent of physicians engaged in this practice.

After my last visit to my parents, I stopped my friend Bill, my father's urologist, in the hospital. Bill was in his greens, harried, obviously between cases.

"Your dad start his radiation treatments?" he asked.

"He hasn't decided what to do."

"What's he waiting for? I'll operate on him if you want—I can get him on the schedule next week. Surgery has a better chance of cure anyway." He was already halfway down the hall.

"Also a better chance of killing him," I said. But nobody heard.

"I was reading here in *Reader's Digest* that people with prostate cancer should have surgery first. Here, read it," my father said.

A couple of weeks had passed since my last pilgrimage to my parents' kitchen. I scanned the article my father handed to me.

"Dad," I said, "The doctor who wrote this is a surgeon. He doesn't know you and your bad heart. I thought we decided against surgery . . ."

"I didn't decide nothing yet!"

"Wait a minute—I thought you and your internist discussed this at the time of the biopsy. He agrees that you're not a surgical candidate at this stage of your life . . ."

He blew into his fist. "My internist is *your* associate! Maybe I should get another opinion."

"Maybe you should," I said.

A week later I was in the middle of office hours; the phone was ringing off the wall. All my exam rooms were full and I was running almost an hour behind. My secretary buzzed me that the urologist was on the phone.

"I just saw your daddy here in my office," he said. "He came in and wanted to know about surgery for his prostate cancer."

"Bill, we've been through this . . ."

"I know, Jerry, I know. While he was here, I called his cardiologist."

"And?"

"He said that if I operate, he himself will file the first malpractice suit."

"So what did you tell my father?"

"I told him he better get started on those radiation treatments and that I would set them up for him starting tomorrow."

"Great! So what'd he say?"

"He said, 'I want to discuss this with my son.' "

"Dad," I said, late that night, "It's time for you to make a decision about this prostate cancer. I hear you saw the urologist today."

"He already called you?"

"Right after you left. So what'd you decide?"

He sat there for a while, his head resting on his arms, elbows on the table.

"Well," he said finally, "your doctor friends are pushing me to have the radiation. Your mother is worried it will be a mess. . . . But this seems to be what you are telling me to do . . ."

"Radiation is a mess, isn't it, Jerry?" my mother said.

"Look, Mom—the issue isn't the mess. We'll get help if he has problems with his bowels. Visiting nurses, aides—whatever it takes. The issue is whether Dad wants to have any treatment at all for this. We can wait and treat him later if he has real problems, or we can use drugs. They're like hormones . . ."

"I'm not taking no hormones!" my father yelled across that checkered, half-century divide.

"Okay, Dad! We don't even have to think about that now. The issue before us is the radiation therapy. Your doctors feel like this has the best chance of cure for you today . . ."

"Even if tomorrow I'm a mess?"

"God, Dad, will you just make a decision on this! It's your body, your life we're talking about here."

"You don't have to raise your voice, Jerry," my mother said. "Your father just wants you to tell him what he should do. You're the doctor in the family, after all."

I took a deep breath. "Have the radiation treatments, Dad," I said, staring at the table.

"So. It'll be on your head," he said.

"Promise me there won't be a mess," my mother pleaded.

When I got home that night, Johnny Carson had just finished his monologue. I plopped down on the bed beside my wife. I heard her tell me to take off my shoes. Then nothing. The screen went blank. White. I remember trying to fight something, then just letting go . . .

I was transported again into the ER. Leslie was frightened; this seizure had lasted longer than the last one. She had called my parents and we were all crowded into the little exam cubicle. My mother dabbed her eyes with a tissue, her mascara running; my father stood off in the corner, looking down, blowing into his hand. Steve was there once again, going over me, checking my reflexes.

"You stop your medicine?" he asked me.

"Of course not! Just check my Dilantin level, give me a bolus if it's low, and sign me the hell out of here!"

"I think you should stay the night," Steve said.

"Listen to the doctor," my mother said.

My father said nothing.

The next morning I was out in time for office hours.

My father underwent a series of radiation treatments. He had some problems: radiation burns on the skin, bouts of bloody diarrhea, some temporary urinary incontinence. It was nothing my family couldn't handle. The cancer has never returned.

A few years back my father and I were sitting together at the kitchen table. I was telling him about my day, jabbering on about a patient I was worried about in intensive care, a woman with a bad stroke and seizures. I was trying to distract him so he would eat the pot roast and potatoes my mother had prepared.

Out of the blue he said, "It's my fault about your seizures. I never should have handed you to that jerky little cousin of your mother's.

At your bris. Right through his arms you went, like a botched hand-off . . ."

I was astonished. My father's face turned white. I reached over and put my hand on his arm.

"I snatched you up from the floor," he went on. "Your eyes rolled back for a second, but I shook you and then you seemed okay, like any baby. I didn't know what could happen so long after . . ." He began to cry.

My poor father. Not only has he forgotten most of the good times between us, he is still haunted by the mistakes—real or imagined—he has made in my upbringing and in his life. Dementias, I have found, are often like this. They rob their sufferers of what is most precious and magnify the fears and paranoia of what remains.

I gently squeezed my father's arm. "Forget it, Dad. I'm fine. I haven't had a seizure in years. You were a wonderful father to me."

That night I watched as he ate his meal and cleaned his plate. I had sat with him at this same table as a boy when he came home late from his long days at the pawnshop. My mother and brother and I would have eaten earlier on those evenings, but I would sit with my father, wait for him to tell me about his day or perhaps about a new bird he'd seen that morning in our yard, or a fishing trip he might be planning. In those days, he did most of the talking. Now I do.

We have never discussed this chapter of my own medical history again. Perhaps he has finally, blissfully, forgotten.

NINE

In 1977 my parents moved to San Antonio. My mother came to work in my medical office. She was fifty-three years old. Until then she had never used a multi-line phone; something as simple as putting a call on "hold" bewildered her. But she was respectful and helpful to all the folks, young and old, who came to the office seeking our help. Over the years, as our practice grew, my mother learned new skills. She was the first to be trained in the use of our computerized billing system; she taught everyone who followed. By the time my mother retired—a forced retirement due to her macular degeneration—she was almost eighty and had worked in my office for twenty-six years. My patients miss her to this day.

During those years my mother worked in the office—keeping the accounts straight, dealing with insurance companies, maintaining friendships with our nurses and techs and secretaries—my father was mostly alone during the weekdays. He read or painted or went to the library. For many years he picked my daughters up from school and brought them back to his house for a snack. He taught them how to draw; they watched TV together. He looked after them with patience and love until our workday was over.

When my mother came home each evening, she and my father usually went out to dinner. He never learned to cook and she was too tired. They never went anywhere fancy: the Luby's cafeteria just a mile away, perhaps the neighborhood Chinese place. One night about seven years ago my mother called me. "There's something wrong with your father," she said.

"What is it, Mom? What happened?"

"I don't know . . . he got lost coming home from Luby's tonight, and I tried to tell him he turned the wrong way but he just blew up at me. We drove around for almost an hour—I didn't say another word—and when we finally got home, he couldn't open the door. I mean, it wasn't like he couldn't find the key. . . . It was like he forgot what to do with the key."

"I'll come over," I said.

When I got to my parents' house, I found my mother sitting in front of the TV in the living room. My father was back in his bedroom, reading.

"Mom," I said, "how long has this been going on?"

"A few months. I didn't want to bother you. I thought he was just being stubborn."

My father didn't hear me coming into his bedroom. He almost never wore his hearing aids.

"Hello, Jerry-boy," he said, looking up. "What are you doing here at this hour?" On the bed next to him was a book of van Gogh paintings; on his chest, Joseph Heller's *Catch-22*. He must have read this a dozen times already.

I pulled up a chair.

"Dad," I said. "Mom told me what happened tonight."

"What happened?" he said.

"You got lost driving home from Luby's."

"That's bullshit," he said. "Your mother's always exaggerating. I took one wrong turn. It was dark."

"Dad, you drove around for an hour—and then you couldn't figure out how to open the front door! We've got to get you checked
out."

"There's nothing wrong with me. Just leave me alone."

His eyes wandered to the book beside him. "This is a good book,
by the way. Here, you take it," he said.

"No, thanks. I've read it—and so have you, by the way."

"Well, my memory's not so good anymore. Every time is like the
first time and I get a chuckle out of it."

"Dad, that's what I'm talking about. Your memory is going, and I
want you to come to the office and see Dr. Galan about it."

"Are you looking for more trouble with me?"

"I just want you to get yourself checked out is all . . ."

"Forget about it," he said.

Most of us don't recognize when our spouses or parents begin to lose
their mental capacities until something dramatic happens. My mother
didn't understand that my father was demented; she believed his
stubbornness and withdrawal were purposeful acts of belligerence
against her. She blamed him for his disability until that night he
couldn't find his way home, couldn't unlock the front door by himself. Adult children are often no different in their lack of insight: We
expect our parents, after all, to be our parents.

The truth is that I suspected my father had been developing a dementia for some time. He was more withdrawn, became easily agitated, especially in social situations. Our conversations were fine—as
long as we kept to superficialities. "How's it going, Dad?" or "How
about this heat!" or "The kids are doing just fine . . ." If I asked anything specific about a book he was reading, his stock answer was "I
haven't gotten that far yet." He stopped watching movies on television. At first I thought it was his hearing and my brother got him one
of those earphone amplifier devices that worked very well—if he remembered to use it. But he mostly tuned in to sports events and game

shows—*Jeopardy* was a favorite—and I was always surprised when he came up with a correct answer. He gave up on programming that required following a plot.

My father certainly had many of the risk factors for dementia: His status as an "old old" man, his lack of higher education, a history of high blood pressure and heart disease, his sedentary lifestyle, and his prior bouts of depression. Add to this his retirement at a relatively early age, his withdrawal from social interactions, and my father had set himself up for cognitive loss in his old age.

And yet there is so much we don't know about the fundamental causes of dementia. After all, my father did spend his sixties and seventies in the pursuit of his art, as solitary an undertaking as this was. He taught himself art history, experimented with painting techniques and produced dozens of canvases, read hundreds of books, wrote piles of letters to his siblings and nephews back in Baltimore. Perhaps my father was just unlucky. Perhaps he was programmed at birth—by nature and early nurture—to mentally self-destruct, destined to eventually lose his personhood from the moment he was delivered from his mother's womb.

My father did come in for a checkup. I knocked on the door of the exam room where my father and Dr. Galan were visiting. I heard them laughing together. When I popped my head in, my father said, "Jerry-boy, what are you doing here?" I didn't know whether he was being sociable and I caught him by surprise or if he'd forgotten that I worked in the same office as Dr. Galan.

"I just stopped in to say hi, Dad. I'll see you later," I said, nodding to my associate.

After his visit, Dr. Galan and I talked.

"Honestly, I don't find too much," he said. "He's oriented and appropriate and has a sense of humor. He had a little trouble with word recall, but that was it. I ordered the usual—some thyroid functions, a vitamin B-12 level. Oh, and your dad agreed to have a brain scan. I think he's okay, though."

"Do you think he's depressed, John?" I asked.

"Not really. He was pretty lively in there. And funny, too." he said.

Dementia is difficult to diagnose in the early stages. Perhaps as many as 95 percent of mild dementia cases are not detected by doctors; even moderate cases may be missed more than 70 percent of the time. Many folks, like my father, can rise to the occasion of an office visit and do very well, especially when their social skills are still intact. Of course, after I relayed to Dr. Galan what had been going on with my dad at home, he was more concerned and glad he had ordered the additional tests. Without this important history—and where is it going to come from if not the family?—a clinician just doesn't have the information needed to consider a diagnosis of dementia.

My father's laboratory tests were all normal for his age. His brain scan showed some organ shrinkage, some hardening of the arteries—nothing unusual for an almost-eighty-year-old man. Indeed, these scan findings were consistent with a diagnosis of dementia, but many folks his age with totally intact cognitive abilities share these sorts of findings. Still, the tests were not a waste of time. We eliminated other possibilities: excess fluid filling the brain ventricles, a tumor, a critically blocked artery, or a collection of blood under the skull bone (perhaps, as can often happen, from a fall no one knew about) pressing on brain matter. Something, perhaps, that was fixable.

Meanwhile, my mother was cooking again most nights. She didn't want to risk going out with my father and getting lost, then having a big fight. During the day he still drove himself around—to the mall, the library, occasionally to the art museum—quite a trek from his usual neighborhood haunts. When he told me about these outings, I expressed my fears. I relayed the story of a man, my patient, who had left his house early in the morning just to go out to his local grocery for some milk. At nightfall they found him, confused and dehydrated, his car driven onto the shoulder of Loop 410, the highway that surrounds the city. He had spent all day circling and circling San Antonio, not knowing where he was or how to exit the highway, until he ran out of gas.

My father only shrugged. "What do you think I am, crazy or something?"

I knew my father shouldn't be driving; he was a danger to himself and others, not to mention my mother when she went out with him. She could no longer drive—especially at night—due to her eyesight.

"What are we going to do about Dad's driving?" my brother and I asked each other. I knew what I had to do, but I dreaded it.

One Sunday afternoon I went over to my parents' house. My father was at the kitchen table working the Jumble. "Dad," I said, "it's a beautiful day. Why don't we take a little ride? Let's go over to Brackenridge Park—maybe we'll see some birds?"

"Yeah, sure," he said. "We haven't been bird-watching together in a long time, have we Jerry-boy?"

He put on his hat, then his jacket—the latest in a series that my mother bought to replace the ones left behind in restaurants or bookstores or the library. We walked out to the driveway.

"Why don't we take your car, Dad?" I said. "I'm almost out of gas."

"Okay," he said.

We stood for a minute on either side of his old Ford Taurus. Most of the paint had flecked off the roof and hood, a consequence of the unforgiving South Texas sun. One of the tires was low. He held the remote car-door opener, turning it over and over in his hand.

"Come on, Dad," I said. "Open the door."

He set the alarm off. The horn blared. He didn't know what to do. I came around, took the keys from him, opened the door, engaged the ignition, and the sound stopped.

"I hate that damn thing," he said.

"Just get in, Dad. Let's go birding."

We started out. My father clutched the steering wheel with both hands, his head barely clearing the top of it. He seemed to have forgotten how to use his rearview mirror. He almost missed the stop sign at the corner and had to slam on the brakes when I yelled about an oncoming car. Ten minutes later—and after two other potentially dangerous incidents—he pulled into the empty parking lot of my medical office.

"I thought we were going bird-watching at Brackenridge Park," I said.

"Oh, yeah," he said. "I forgot. I just sort of automatically come over here. I guess from all the times I used to pick up your mother."

"Dad, you shouldn't be driving anymore. You almost got us killed three times. I want you to tell me you'll give up the car."

"You're exaggerating," he said. "Your mother put you up to this, didn't she?" His knuckles were white, still gripping the wheel.

"Dad, please. This isn't about Mom. How would you feel if you injured or killed someone?"

"I've never had an accident in my life and I've been driving a helluva long time, a lot longer than you."

"There's a time to stop, just like there's a time to start," I said. "And your time has come."

"I've had a car since I was seventeen years old . . . I'll be a prisoner in my own house . . ."

"Mike and I will take you anywhere you want to go, you know that. We can even hire someone to drive you around. There's a van that will pick you up and take you to senior activities . . ."

"I'm not sitting around with a bunch of old people," he said.

"Dad," I said, my tone softening, "we'll work all this out. Many people your age give up driving, and life goes on . . ."

He sat there, his head drooped onto his chest, his hands still on the wheel. "Here, you drive home," he said, and he opened his door.

"Don't you want to go down to the park?"

"Just take me home."

The next weekend my brother sold the old Taurus. My father was angry with us all for about a month, avoided me when I came over for a visit. He feigned sleep or wouldn't come out of his bedroom.

One night, not too long after, we all went out to dinner together to celebrate my mother's birthday. I ordered beers for me and my father. "Dad," I asked him, "do you miss not having the car?"

He put down his half-empty mug and stared into it for a while. "I guess we did the right thing," he said.

TEN

There is a chart storage room in my office building that is the size of a two-car garage. It's a quiet space, to me a solemn space. The walls are fifteen feet high and lined with steel shelving, floor to ceiling. On these shelves sit file boxes and in these boxes are individual patient charts; I estimate fifteen thousand or so. These charts contain my hand-written or voice-transcribed notes on the one quarter million face-to-face patient encounters I have made in my years as a practicing doctor.

I have never discarded a patient's chart, even though by law I am only obligated to keep them for seven years. In these charts I have documented the complaints, concerns, fears, physical findings, laboratory and X-ray results, consultative opinions, and often—too often—the suffering and demise of hundreds of my patients, some of whom I knew for decades. These are the men and women who have entrusted themselves to my care, who have told me their medical stories, their life stories. They have allowed me to touch and probe their bodies and draw blood from their veins. They have, in their trust of me, undergone countless deeper probings, patiently suffered discomfort and pain and indignities in the belief that I would ease their travails, calm their fears, reassure them, treat their sicknesses, and sometimes even save their lives.

They are my family now, and though many of them are gone, if I hold any single chart in my hand and leaf through the pages, I remember each and every one. As with any family, I remember some with more fondness than others. Yes, there were some who didn't like me; maybe I reminded them too much of their old doctor. Or not enough. Some who didn't like what I had to tell them about their health; some who took my advice and still didn't get well. There were those who didn't like my candor, or perhaps those for whom I was not candid enough. Some disliked me because after they put me on a pedestal of their own making, they found out I was only human. And, yes, some I did fail. Still, many hundreds have continued to come year after year, decade after decade. They are from all walks of life and are mostly old now. They trust me. And my feelings toward them are akin to how I feel about my own parents. If I say that in some way I love them, well, I will be scorned by my colleagues as being paternalistic and overly subjective. Maybe even a little crazy.

I have been married to my second wife, Lee, for nine years. When we first met, she was a successful lawyer in Charleston, South Carolina. We had a long-distance courtship for a while. She wanted me to move back East, leave Texas, and retire. She was well paid. She would support us. She loved Charleston, had many friends there. We could buy a little house on Folly Beach, on the marsh side. I would awake to the sounds of red-winged blackbirds calling from the spartina grass, spend my days watching great blue herons and snowy egrets wade the shallows. I could write, and if I wanted— only if I wanted—I could do some part-time doctoring in a clinic somewhere. She knew everyone; opportunities would arise.

I thought about leaving my patients, my parents—but only for a minute. Well, maybe longer than a minute. When the time came, my wife-to-be moved west.

One recent morning, before light, my alarm clock went off. I fumbled with it in my half-sleep, pushed in the button, but the beeping didn't stop. I realized finally that it was only 5 A.M., two hours before I usually rise, and that the sound was coming from some other object on my nightstand. Besides the clock, there is a telephone, a pager, and a cell phone, all the implements I lay out every night in case someone needs me. For over thirty years I have lived my life in San Antonio waiting for the next call.

My cell phone was beeping, a policeman on the other end. The answering service patched him through to me.

"Are you the doctor?" he asked.

"Yes," I said. I was fully awake now, my heart pounding. Besides hundreds of sick and aging patients, I have grown children out there in the world, and my frail, elderly parents.

"This is Officer Garza with the SAPD. Do you have a patient, Nancy Winters?"

"Yes. . . . What's wrong?" I have known Nancy for over twenty years. She's my mother's age, over eighty. Two years ago I diagnosed her ovarian cancer. With surgery and radiation and chemotherapy she has done remarkably well and still lives independently, alone, her husband having died a few years ago. She is one of a group of women, all friends, who are my patients, though their number is dwindling. Sometimes I see them dining out together in a seafood place we all frequent and I go over to their table. We laugh about how long they've been coming to me, about how we are growing old together.

"We entered her home at the request of her daughter, who has been unable to get in touch with her. Found her on the floor by the bed. She's been dead a while. Daughter doesn't want an autopsy."

This is, of course, why he is calling me. If I can explain with reasoned medical confidence why my patient died, he will tell the medical examiner and perhaps avoid the otherwise mandatory investigation.

"Look," I said, "I just saw her last week. She has metastatic cancer. Tell the ME to call me. She doesn't need an autopsy if there's nothing else suspicious."

"No, nothing here, Doctor. I'll note what you said in my report. Thanks."

After I hung up, I thought about Nancy, about how she might have died. If the cancer had invaded her aorta, she might have hemorrhaged into her abdominal cavity. Or perhaps she had a stroke or a heart attack. However her end came, she went quickly. Now she wouldn't have to make that move she was dreading—from this city and all her remaining friends, to live with her daughter, a decision being urged on her by concerned children. At her last visit to me we talked about this move, about the fact that her time was limited and how she was torn between making things easier on her children and living an independent life as long as possible.

"Nancy," I told her, "this is a tough decision, I know . . . but it's getting to be time."

"I know you're right, Doctor," she said. "Soon. I'll decide soon."

She wasn't ready then and I pushed no further.

After the policeman's call, I wondered if I should notify her friends but decided that her daughter would want to do this. I also wondered if there was anything else I could have done, might have picked up, to have extended her life a bit more. Had she complained of any unusual pains at her visit? Did I remember to ask if there had been any change in her stools?

How we each will die—especially when we are old and plagued by chronic illness—is unpredictable. Every caring, compulsive physician constantly reexamines the details of any case that has an unexpected outcome, a plot twist at the end of the story. This time, in Nancy's case, I decided that my conscience was clear.

I was tired, but I couldn't go back to sleep even though I had the day off. I tried to get back into a novel I had begun reading the night before but couldn't concentrate. My appetite was off. I went about the morning, ticking things from my perpetual to-do list. The mindless items: changing the air-conditioner filters, sweeping out the garage. I had very little to say, didn't want to be the one to answer the phone. Late in the afternoon Lee asked me what was wrong.

"It's nothing," I said. She pressed. "I'm just tired," I said. And then later, when she asked again, I answered, "I don't know."

Finally I realized what was wrong. "Nancy Winters died. That's what the call was." She hadn't heard; she has already developed an ability in our young marriage to sleep right through the rings and beeps and my one-sided conversations.

I told her about Nancy, her years with me—her illness and struggles, her sense of humor, her pride and independence. I reminded her that she met Nancy once at the Sea Island restaurant.

"I don't know why I feel bad, though," I said. "I did everything I could for her. You'd think after so many years of this, after so many losses, it would just roll off."

"It's okay to be sad," Lee said. "That's how you mourn."

Of course, I know this. Kübler-Ross and the stages of grief—denial, anger, bargaining, depression, acceptance. All that. I've repeated them to countless husbands and wives, sons and daughters—the families that remain—over decades now. I can say them in my sleep, recite them as mantra. I only hope I have helped the families of my patients more than I have helped myself.

In my doctoring life, I have tried to follow the example of my best medical school and residency mentors. Even so, I have made mistakes that haunt me to this day. I have tried my best to learn from them. Even the mistakes I have made being a son to my father ultimately made me a better doctor to my patients. My father would appreciate hearing me say this and I would love nothing more than to tell him, but it is too late.

After I earned my medical degree, I trained in an academic internal medicine program. For every conceivable medical question, someone smarter or more experienced than I had an answer. The crush of patients—this inexorable profusion of the sick and dying—always had something to teach me, to teach us.

I was, in those years, in a constant state of "*dis*-ease"; worrying about what I didn't know, trying to protect myself from the constant losses over which I presided. I tried not to allow my starched white coat to become my personal armor against human suffering. Back then I had no idea that I would be in this state of *dis*-ease for the rest of my medical career.

But, more and more, this old, familiar *dis*-ease of mine is being supplanted by another. I am heartsick over what is happening to medical care in America. You will have read the accounts or heard the stories: Medical scientists violating ethical rules in their sometimes questionable relationships with industry and pharmaceutical company–funded research in order to keep the grant money flowing. Physicians in private practice falling over each other, crassly competing, trying to put into place the next money-making technological gimmick: fat suckers, vein zappers, bodily enhancements of every imaginable sort. How many physicians do we need to train to do eyelid rejuvenation, liposuction, and breast implants? Just open up your local Yellow Pages and turn to "Physicians." It is a sobering experience for someone like me, heavily involved in the primary care of the aged, that I have trouble locating a plastic surgeon willing to bring his skills to bear in helping heal a pressure ulcer in a bed-bound, Medicaid-funded nursing-home patient.

A growing number of my primary care colleagues no longer see Medicare patients. One of them told me: "It just takes so long for them to dress and undress and climb off and on the table from their walkers and wheelchairs. . . . It just doesn't pay." Another makes sure he asks each elder, on admission to the hospital, whether she has executed an "advance directive" before he ever probes her chief complaint or puts his stethoscope into his ears. That way he can write the "Do Not Resuscitate" order in her chart first thing.

And what managed care has wrought, what our profession has allowed to occur on its watch: doctor-patient relationships reduced to corporate contracts, the forced dissolution of bonds forged over years of clinical encounters, the implementation of perverse bonus systems which reward physicians for *not* giving care, the substitution of a provider-consumer commodity model in the place of a noble calling.

Yet, despite my concerns about medicine's evolution from a cottage industry into a corporate business model, I have only wonderful things to say about my fellow physicians who do their best, day in and day out, to care for their patients, my patients. Where would I be, how could I begin to do my job without the help of the stalwart cardiologist who for decades has dragged himself out of bed in the dead of night to meet me in the ER, my patient in the throes of an acute myocardial infarction, to whisk her into the cath lab to open a blocked artery? Or the cardiothoracic surgeon who must be awakened next should the procedure fail and the patient need bypass surgery? And my old friend, the orthopedist: How many times did I call him needing an emergency hip procedure after one of my osteoporotic ladies fell and fractured her trochanter? What we have witnessed together over the course of our long careers is this: Our profession—from the most prestigious medical academies to your corner doc-in-the-box—has, in too many arenas, abdicated its patient advocacy role.

When I was a medical student, a professor of internal medicine wrote in his evaluation of my performance: "His concern for his patients is of the highest order." He didn't say I was the brightest student he ever had, because I wasn't; he didn't comment on my knowledge of the medical literature; he didn't say my skills as a diagnostician were advanced, because they weren't. At that early stage of my training I thought he had slighted me. But he knew what "good" doctors come to know: that the only quality that counts in the long run is the degree to which a physician cares about his patient. It is caring that drives one to be cautious, to be compulsively thorough, to be restless in the face of conflicting data or anxious until a prescribed course of therapy elicits a definite positive response.

The family physician and poet William Carlos Williams once described his connection with his patients in this way:

> *"I lost myself in the very properties of their minds: for the mo-*
> *ment at least I actually became* them . . . *so that when I detached*
> *myself from them . . . it was as though I were reawakening from a*
> *sleep."*

Imperfect as I am, I want to do the best I can for my patients, as if
they were members of my own family. I do not hold myself apart;
what happens to them can happen to me, *will* happen to me. We are
all in this life—for as long as it may last—together. I will sign the
guest books at their funerals and stand in the rain at their burials.

From my years as a geriatrician and now as the son of an old, old
man, I recognize this inescapable truth: Our parents will become
our children if they live long enough. I don't mean this in a conde-
scending way. The fact is that almost half of our parents will develop a significant dementia before they die; most of the others
will be debilitated with cancer or heart disease in the end. Perhaps
if we looked upon our elderly as people we need to care for as they
once cared for us, we would be kinder to them. They will—almost
all of them—become dependent upon us, our stronger arms, our
acts of gentleness and compassion. We will arrange for their meals,
pay their bills, take them to their doctor visits, sit by their bedsides
at the hospital, in the nursing home. Be present for them at the end.

"You look tired, Jerry-boy," my father said to me a while back. It was
one of his "good" days. We were sitting on the patio, watching the
cardinals and blue jays flit to and from the bird feeder.
    "It's just been a long day, Dad."
    "Maybe you should retire," he said.

"I'm too young for that. Besides, what would I do?"

"We could go fishing. Remember, we used to do that? It's been a long time . . ."

"Who'll take care of my patients then, Dad?"

"You're not the only doctor in the world," he said.

He can still surprise me, my old father.

ELEVEN

When my daughter Betsy was to be married, just a few months after my father stopped driving, he refused to attend the ceremony.

My mother was furious. "You won't go to your granddaughter's wedding? What's the matter with you?"

I tried to be patient. "Dad, this is a once-in-a-lifetime event. Some of your Baltimore family will be there."

"I just don't think I can make it," he said.

"What are you talking about? I'll pick you and Mom up, drive you to the wedding, we'll stay a couple of hours, and I'll bring you back home. Nothing to it."

"No," he said.

"Dad, Betsy's other grandfather will be there wearing oxygen. He's so short of breath he can barely talk, but he wouldn't miss the wedding for the world."

"I just can't make it," he said.

I have a photograph of my father and my first-born daughter. Betsy is perhaps a year old and my father as old as I am now. They are seated in the brown corduroy rocking chair my first wife, Leslie, and I bought—our only new furniture at the time—to nurse our daughter when she came into this world.

Betsy is sitting in my father's lap, on his right thigh. They are both pointing at me, the cameraman, their left arms extended. "She's a leftie, just like me!" my father said when he first saw this picture.

My father loved all of his grandchildren, but Betsy had the distinction of being his first and she had, besides his handedness, his artist's eye for drawing and color and composition. Many times when I picked up my daughters from his house during the years he took care of them after school, he brandished a drawing Betsy had made. "Look at this," he said. "The girl's got real talent here."

On his seventieth birthday my family put together an album for my father. It took us months to complete. We sorted and chose photos of him from throughout his life. Many I had enlarged and colorized. Leslie inscribed aphorisms from *Bartlett's* in her calligraphic script:

"*Age does not make us childish, as they say. It only finds us true children still.*" (Goethe)

"*For age is opportunity no less than youth itself.*" (Longfellow)

"*It is impossible to please all of the world and one's father.*" (de la Fontaine)

My father was overcome when we presented this album to him. Tears rolled down his cheeks as he lifted each leaf and studied the photographs: his mother, sisters and brothers when they were young and vigorous; a dashing image of him in the Army Air Corps posed with his Speed Graphic; his young bride at their wedding; his two sons growing up again before his eyes as he turned the pages.

"This is the most wonderful present anyone has ever given me," he told us. And then, as if he didn't really deserve it, he added, "But you really made this for yourselves, didn't you? I mean you'll have this for a long time after I'm gone, won't you?" He couldn't believe anyone would ever go to this much trouble just for him.

Our daughters each wrote him a letter that we pasted into this album. Emily wrote:

2/1/89

Dear Grandpa,

Here is a letter to thank you for always being there for me. I appreciate it more than anything in the world. I hope you know that, but if you don't, I'm telling you now.

Whenever Betsy or I were sick you were always there for us. You let us stay in your house, on your couch, and put up with our fevers, our coughs, our throw up, our sneezes and our aches and pains. You made us tea and soup and always made sure we were as comfortable as could be. I don't know what we'd do if your kind heart wasn't there for us.

How in the world could you stand picking us up from school all those years? And always making sure there was something for our snack? Oh, not to mention the dancing lessons for a year. Grandpa, you're just too much! Every Thursday for a whole summer you took us somewhere. I remember going to museums and lunch with you.

I love you, Grandpa.

How could my father now refuse to attend Betsy's wedding? I had a flash of anger at him myself—which I suppressed—even though I understood what he could not express. This demented man, living out his remaining years quietly with his wife—the TV and visits from his close family his only source of stimulation—was now unable to interact with the busy world all of us take for granted. He imagined the crowd, hundreds of people whose names he didn't know or couldn't remember, the platters of food, the flowers, the conversation and laughter assaulting his hearing aids, the noise of a band amplified by loudspeakers, the sight of his once-small granddaughter—the child he remembered—walking down the aisle with a strange man and off into another life: These scenes as he imagined them frightened him more than the specter of his own death.

Betsy didn't fully understand. She and her sister had been off in college and grad school for the past eight years. They spoke with their grandfather once in a while over the phone, stopped in for brief visits at holidays. Their interactions were superficial: *Hi and how are you and I love you and good-bye.* Of course she knew her grandfather was aging, becoming more frail, but his face always lit up when he saw her. "Remember when I used to give you drawing lessons after school?" he said, his own memories flooding back at the sight of her. "We sure had a good time in those days, didn't we?"

"Dad," she asked me. "What's with Grandpa? Is he mad at me? I just don't understand why he won't come to my wedding." I had yet to make it clear to her what was really going on. It was time all of us admitted it: that what my father had was a progressive, degenerative neurological disease.

"Grandpa has Alzheimer's," I said. It was the first time I named his disease out loud to a member of my family or even to myself. "It's going to get worse."

There are multiple causes of dementia—the loss of cognitive function—that half of us will develop if we live long enough. Alzheimer's disease is responsible for perhaps as many as 70 percent of the cases. This slowly progressive disease may take from five to twenty years to fully run its course, depending on the age and health of the patient at the onset. Currently, there are five million patients with this disease in America today. A conservative estimate of the cost to care for them is $100 billion annually. By 2050—if no medical breakthroughs reduce the incidence of Alzheimer's dementia in our country—there will be between eleven and eighteen million people with this condition, costing Medicare a trillion dollars each year.

There are other causes of dementia. Vascular dementia, a consequence of cerebrovascular disease or hardening of the arteries, is often associated with hypertension, heart disease, strokes, diabetes, smoking, and elevated cholesterol levels. Indeed, almost certainly, my father likely has a combination of vascular dementia and Alzheimer's—a so-called mixed dementia. Subtle variations in clinical patterns exist between the various dementias, but as a practical matter, for families dealing with the manifestations in a loved one, the exact distinctions between them are less important than the overwhelming effects of the condition itself.

Most of us—beginning even in middle age—feel we are more forgetful than we once were. If we were to undergo standardized mental status testing at this age—the Mini Mental State Examination (MMSE) is a commonly administered test—we would probably achieve a perfect score of 30. The examiner asks a set of questions to determine a subject's orientation to time and place, tests his ability to recall three simple words immediately and then a few minutes later, checks his skill at rudimentary arithmetic, his ability to name common objects, repeat a stock phrase, perform a series of straightforward but consecutive tasks, tests him on a brief reading and writing sample, and his ability to draw a geometric figure, such as a polygon.

We recognize now that Alzheimer's disease (AD) has a preclinical phase that may be tough to diagnose. MMSE scores, if measured in this phase, will be above 25, and although close family members might notice a change, the patient is still functioning at a high level. At the time of my father's prostate cancer diagnosis he was already in this phase of his illness.

By the time one has had AD for one to three years, the disease is said to be in its early or mild impairment stage. Patients may experience problems with dates, naming objects, recent recall. They may begin to socially withdraw, have difficulty managing their finances, become more irritable. They are losing what is called executive function—the ability to organize and carry out sequential tasks, essential to accomplishing activities such as paying bills, shopping for groceries, or planning a meal. Their judgment is lacking. My father has passed through this stage; he was in it when we took his car away because he was getting lost.

Two to eight years into the disease patients become moderately impaired. That's where we are now with Dad. He is disoriented to place and time, is unable to learn anything new, can no longer make the simplest calculations. He sometimes has delusions and hallucinations, frequent bouts of agitation and anxiety and depression. He needs help to dress and groom himself.

If he lives long enough to reach the severe stage of the disease—six to twelve years—here is how he will be: Even his distant past memories will be gone; he will be unable to speak intelligibly or even sign his name. He will wear diapers. He will stop eating and lose his ability to speak and walk. Eventually he will die. I only hope that something takes him before he reaches this stage.

Perhaps you are thinking that your spouse is exhibiting the early signs of Alzheimer's disease. Or your Mom or Dad. Perhaps you yourself. Do you really want to know? What should you do? Does it make any difference to try to find out as soon as possible? These are hard questions, and until very recently I didn't push my patients who showed the early signs of AD to do anything other than keep active physically and mentally—common-sense advice that is still the cornerstone of dementia management. I've always recommended the basic evaluation to rule out the few treatable causes of dementia: underlying diseases, fluid and electrolyte disorders, drug effects and interactions, thyroid problems, vitamin B-12 deficiency, incubating syphilis, brain tumors or bleeds, hydrocephalus, and depression which can closely mimic AD in its earlier phases.

What about "screening examinations" to detect Alzheimer's in its earliest stages? This is still quite controversial. The Alzheimer's Association endorses public awareness programs but has not yet recommended community assessment of memory problems by physicians using formal mental status testing. Because there is one important caveat here: A positive screen is only an indication for further testing. It does not necessarily mean that a patient definitely has Alzheimer's disease.

These screening recommendations are evolving because there is some hope today that new drugs may, individually or in combination, slow the progression of Alzheimer's disease. Drugs like donepezil inhibit an enzyme, cholinesterase, and increase the amount of acetylcholine—an important neurotransmitter—available in the brain. Memantine blocks a different excitatory neurotransmitter channel affecting available levels of glutamate in areas of the brain that appear to be damaged in AD. Recent studies suggest that perhaps the use of cholinesterase inhibitors in combination with drugs such as memantine may be helpful in the later stages of AD.

Note that I did not say these drugs *cure* Alzheimer's disease. There is no cure. Patients continue to progress with their AD, albeit at a slower rate. Families can manage their loved ones at home longer and perhaps postpone the need for institutionalization.

My father, at his doctor's suggestion, tried these drugs. They did not help him, and he developed the uncommon but intolerable side effects of nausea and increased agitation. But the drugs do help some patients, and the evidence seems to show that the earlier medications are started in the AD process, the slower the inevitable decline will be. Thankfully, AD is the focus of much scientific research and there are other drugs coming along, therapies aimed more directly at the pathological brain processes of AD and the products of the genes responsible, such as the accumulation of abnormal proteins seen under the microscope in diseased organs.

But for now, families with loved ones like my father are just muddling through, trying to take things as they come, one day at time.

Betsy and Art were married surrounded by their family and friends. Grandpa Leonard stayed at home with a health-care aide. The bride and groom, dressed in their wedding finery, came afterward to say their hellos and good-byes.

I have forgiven my father for refusing to come to the wedding because I understand how difficult all this was for him. At that time I was a grown man, fifty-two years old, a father of adult children, a doctor—but I must admit that my forgiveness did not come soon enough in my life with my dad. It took his becoming an old, old man—demented and bereft of his memories—for me to understand that my love for him now must be unconditional, just as his love for me once was.

A few months later the photo album with all the traditional wedding scenes arrived in the mail. There was Betsy walking down the aisle, serene and lovely, then beaming at the camera after the ceremony, feeding Art a piece of wedding cake. I couldn't wait to show my father the photos. He leafed through a page or two. He stared at Betsy, pointed his finger at a close-up of her face.

"Who is that?" he asked.

TWELVE

My parents don't drive anymore: my father because he cannot find his way home, my mother because she can't see. My father secludes himself in his bedroom, turning the pages of a book he's "read" a dozen times. The television blares in the living room—I can hear it before I open the front door. My mother sits with her face a foot from the screen.

They live like this, waiting for a visit from one of their sons. In this they are not alone. So many of our senior citizens sit day after day with nothing better to do than stare, benumbed, into television screens. When they can no longer safely stay in their own homes, we warehouse them in unimaginative institutional settings. Their children are often scattered across the continent, busy with their own lives, working hard to make ends meet, doing their best to be good parents to their own kids. They call their aging parents once a week, visit once or twice a year. These sons and daughters—my boomer brethren—may be completely unaware that Dad is sliding into dementia, that Mom can no longer see to prepare her meals. Then there is a crisis; we are forced to act and make decisions, all too often with incomplete information, without enough time to investigate options.

It doesn't have to be this way. It shouldn't be this way.

How I wish we in America thought differently about our elders. We are all part of a living chain. Each of us in our own family is valuable and should be valued. Perhaps if we can learn to value our parents as they age we can shed some of the fear we ourselves feel as we grow older. My cohort of boomers, always generating controversy, can by our own example change our culture's negative perception of the elderly. We have a slim window of opportunity to transform America before our Golden Years crush us. What a difference we can make before we go.

Helga and Fritz Steiner found their way to me when they were in their late seventies. Fritz had been in the real-estate business and was now comfortably retired in San Antonio. The Steiners had a daughter, Minna, who had long since moved away to California. She rarely visited her parents.

"She's busy with her law practice and her children," Helga explained.

Fritz and Helga had many of the usual problems of the old old. Fritz was fifty pounds overweight with high blood pressure and high cholesterol; Helga had arthritis. They came in together for their appointments. We three sat in the exam room talking, exchanging jokes—Fritz was a great storyteller—before we got down to the business at hand. He always answered for his wife, seemed in control of every situation. I could see why he had been so successful in business.

Helga was a shy, quiet woman. She spoke with a German accent and smiled whenever I managed to dredge up a word or two from my high school classes: "*Wie geht es Ihnen?*" I would say, or "*Guten Tag.*"

One day, Helga came in with a painful rash. The red pustules covered the left side of her face and extended down her neck and upper back. I recognized this as a classic case of shingles, a reactivation of the chicken pox virus that had lain dormant in her nerve ganglia ever since she'd contracted the illness as a young girl. At the time Helga came to me, antiviral therapies were not yet available; nor was the shingles vaccine. Treatment was limited to a short course of cortisone and medications to relieve pain.

Within a few weeks Helga's rash had cleared up, but she continued to experience intense pain. This syndrome of continued pain in the region where the chicken pox rash had initially erupted is called post-herpetic neuralgia. Usually with time and the use of pain-blocking medications, the sensation gradually dissipates, but Helga's searing pain was unremitting. She had the worst post-herpetic neuralgia I had ever seen.

I tried everything. I put her in the hospital for a thorough medical evaluation to make sure she didn't have an underlying disease process or a malignancy, conditions that can affect the body's immune system and allow the reactivation of the varicella virus. My neurology consultants and I looked at her brain and neck and spine and sinuses, searching for evidence of a pinched nerve, a slipped disc, a tumor lurking somewhere, pressing on some vital structure. We found nothing.

I put Helga on pain medications, muscle relaxants, sleeping pills, finally resorting to narcotic analgesics. Only when she managed to drift off to sleep was she pain free. The chronic pain and the drugs killed Helga's appetite. She lost twenty pounds. Of course she was depressed—who wouldn't be?—and I sent her to a psychiatrist who prescribed even more medications. Eventually I agreed to a last-ditch attempt at relief and allowed a neurosurgeon to cut a number of nerve fibers in Helga's neck. This failed as well.

As they became unable to travel or entertain or even leave their home except for doctor appointments, Fritz and Helga's world collapsed. During our visits, Fritz often turned to me and said, "Do me a favor, Doctor, give our daughter Minna a call. Let her know how bad off Helga is." I spoke to Minna on the phone many times at his request.

I began visiting the Steiners at home every couple of weeks. They lived far from the medical center, but whenever I knew I was going to be in their area of town I'd stop by. The house was dark, the shades and curtains always drawn. Figurines, silver pieces, knick-knacks covered every flat, undusted surface. Helga perked up when I visited. She'd get out of bed and come into the living room. Fritz told the old stories. We'd laugh together, drink tea, eat ginger cookies.

"Fritz," I said to him, as he showed me out, "Helga does better with people around. I'm going to call a home health agency, have nurses and therapists and social workers come by. Maybe there's an adult day-care center nearby. You both need to get out of this house."

"Don't you dare call anyone," he said. "I don't want anybody coming and going through here. There's a lot of valuable stuff sitting out around here . . ."

"Fritz, you and Helga need some help—you especially. You can't go on like this!"

"If you want to do something, call my daughter."

"Minna, I'm really worried about your parents," I told her on the phone that night. "They're virtual shut-ins. Your dad won't let me get any help for them. Maybe if you come for a visit you can talk him into it . . ."

There was a long silence on the line before she answered. "I love my parents," she said, "but I have longstanding issues with my father. He's a bully and my mother lets him get away with it. I couldn't wait to get out of that house."

"Minna, they're old and sick now. Your mother may be dying of loneliness. They're just barely hanging on . . ."

"Look, Doctor, I care about them, but it's so hard for me to get away on short notice."

"Just come for a weekend. Your father asks me all the time to call you. I know they'd both be boosted by your presence and then maybe together we can convince them to make some changes . . . I'm worried something will happen."

"I'll see what I can arrange."

Two weeks went by. I called Fritz and asked him if he'd heard from Minna. She hadn't called.

"Why don't you come by on Friday?" he said.

"I can't. I'm taking the family down to Rockport for the weekend."

"Why don't you stop by on your way out of town? It's been a while since I've seen your daughters," he said.

"If I get finished early enough I'll do that. Otherwise, I'll get over there next week for sure."

Rockport is a charming town on the Texas coast. With its live-oak groves, marshes, and shallow bays, it's a birder's paradise, and I loved spending time there with my family on the rare weekends we could get away. We packed the station wagon early that Friday morning and dropped the children at school. My wife and I raced around all day, solved one problem after another, always the squeeze-ins at the end of the week. Finally we were finished and signed out to our weekend coverage. We picked up our kids, who were waiting impatiently for us at Grandpa's house.

It was already rush hour and we were stuck in traffic on I-10. "I should stop off and check on the Steiners," I said. My daughters groaned from the backseat.

"I hate going over there," Emily said.

"Yeah," Betsy piped in. "It's so dark and depressing in that house."

"Are they sick?" Leslie asked.

"They're the same," I said. "It was going to be more or less a social call."

"Can't we skip it today? As it is, we won't make it to Rockport until almost nine. We'll be starving by then."

"Okay," I said. "I'll check on them next week."

My kids cheered.

The next morning, Saturday, I got up early and walked along Aransas Bay, up Fulton Beach Road and out to Live Oak Point. I saw a few birds: a black and white warbler, a couple of Eastern kingbirds, a purple martin. The spring migration was in its earliest stage. On Sunday morning I sat sipping my coffee, watching the news coming in from Corpus Christi. A reporter described a murder-suicide in the Steiners' neighborhood of San Antonio. Two elderly people, a husband and wife, had been taken to University Hospital. I looked at my wife.

"We've got to go back," I said.

Nearly twenty Americans die each week in homicide-suicides. These numbers are up tenfold since 1988. Desperate acts, arising out of loneliness, isolation, and depression, they are carried out most often by elderly domineering husbands who find themselves in a caregiving role, in situations that have little chance of improving. I am afraid these numbers are only going to increase as our society continues to age.

Fritz shot Helga in the head and then shot himself. He died instantly. She lingered on in an ICU for a week before she succumbed. Perhaps he thought he was putting her out of her misery.

I did talk to Minna afterward although I never did meet her. "Well, you told me you thought something would happen, Doctor," she said. "And it did."

I have been a surrogate son for many of my patients over the years. I have asked hundreds of thousands of questions—millions by now—of the folks who have come to me for care. In posing enough questions I usually get to the bottom of the problem and can help. These days, because of increasing suicide and murder-suicide rates, doctors who care for the oldest among us are encouraged to ask their homebound patients questions we would never have asked before.

"Fritz," I would ask today, "do you have a gun?"

THIRTEEN

When I was a boy, my father read me the books that had enthralled him when he was young, especially the Jack London novels, *The Call of the Wild* and *White Fang*.

"Did you ever have a dog when you were a boy?" I asked him.

"I was always bringing home strays or injured puppies," he said. "Granny never let me keep them. It costs money to have a dog and we didn't have much back then."

I was seven years old. Week after week, on my way home from Liberty School #64, I stopped to watch the black and white and brown mutts roll around in the sawdust behind the pet store window. They wagged their tails and licked my fingers when I went inside to play with them. "Four dollars each," said the lady behind the counter. A fortune.

"Dad, can we get a dog?"

By then we were living on Forest Park Avenue, in a two-story Cape Cod with a full basement. The house sat, one among a block of similar homes, on a rise just across the avenue from an eighteen-hole municipal golf course. The green expanse, with its woodland roughs and ponds, beckoned to a young boy, especially one who dreamed of having a dog by his side.

"I really want a dog, Dad," I said. "They cost four dollars at the pet store."

"Do you have four dollars?" he asked.

"No," I said.

"Do you know anything about taking care of a dog?"

"No."

"Go to the library and check out some books about dogs," he said. "Learn how to care for one first."

This assignment seemed easy enough. I loved the library.

"Okay," I said. "But what about the four dollars?"

"You'll have to save up the money," he said.

"I never get any money except when Grandma gives me pennies or dimes. I'll never have four dollars!"

"It's time for you to have an allowance, Jerry-boy." He reached into his pocket, fished out a quarter, and pushed it across the table. "Every week I'll give you a quarter. Save it for the movies, comic books, baseball cards, whatever you want. Save it up for a dog. It's your money."

I remember taking that quarter up to my room, finding an empty metal Band-Aid box, and dropping it in. That first coin made a hollow sound, but four months later the container, heavy with silver, held enough money to buy a dog.

"I've saved up four dollars," I said the evening he gave me the sixteenth installment of my allowance. I emptied the coins onto the kitchen table, made four neat stacks of four quarters each. "Can we go get a dog now?"

"Not yet," he said. In this fifty-year-old memory I realize that my father seemed uneasy, unsure. My mother was at the kitchen sink, the faucet running, her hands in dishwater. It was winter; we had just finished dinner and already it was dark outside.

"But, Dad, you promised . . ."

"You need to save more money. The dog will need to eat, you know."

I left the quarters on the table and went up to my room. My father did not read to me that night. As I fell asleep, I heard my parents arguing. The next morning the golf course across the street had filled with snow, deep drifts glistening like the Klondike I imagined when my father read to me from London's books.

School was cancelled that day; my father was late coming home from the store because of the bad weather. My mother had his dinner on the table for him as if she knew he'd be in a hurry to eat. I picked at my food. I couldn't look at my father.

After the meal he said, "Let's go get your dog now, Jerry-boy." He was smiling; he looked over at my mother and she was smiling, too. I retrieved my Band-Aid box with its cache of quarters.

I will never forget that night. The snow started again just as we left the house, the temperature dropping. My father drove slowly, deliberately. There were few cars on the streets, many others stuck in drifts along the roadsides. As we approached the pet store I could see that the lights were off.

"Dad, we'll have to come back tomorrow . . ."

"We're not going to the pet store," he said. He pulled a newspaper ad out of his pocket. "There's a family in Towson who raises collies; they have a new litter for sale."

"A collie?" I said. I watched Lassie every week on television. A beautiful, smart collie. A friend, a protector. "Really, Dad?"

"When I was a boy, we had a neighbor down the street who had a collie. Duke was his name. He and I had a lot of good times together . . ."

We got our own Duke that night. The pick of the litter. The Logans had been raising collies for years, award-winning dogs. I watched my father hand over two twenty-dollar bills in exchange for this gangly, trembling animal I gathered in my arms. I felt elated—and worried. I knew this was a lot of money to pay for a dog, but I was not going to let go of him.

On the journey home the roads were iced over. We inched along. The hard pull up Cold Spring Lane took forever. The old

DeSoto chugged a foot, then slid back a few inches. Cars lay splayed in all directions, nosed into drifts and into each other. Heavy snow obscured the traffic signals. Duke trembled, then peed on me. I didn't say anything. My father was hunched over the wheel; he knew how to steer into the skid, gingerly use the brake, downshift into the turns.

This was our own grand adventure: braving the winter elements together, bound by one purpose. It is a story we tell each other, even now. Even as his dementia progresses, if I say, "Dad, remember that night we went to get Duke? That blizzard?" he perks up, begins to recount this distant episode.

"I wanted the pick of the litter . . . I must have been crazy to go out in that storm."

When we finally made it home that night, my mother was frantic. She had put newspapers down on the kitchen floor. That was their deal: Duke could stay in the kitchen for now and then the basement when he got bigger, but he wouldn't have access to the rest of the house, even though the sofa in the living room was encased in plastic slipcovers.

My little brother was asleep upstairs in his crib. I was excited but exhausted. I hugged my parents, thanked them over and over for letting me have this dog. Duke peed on the kitchen floor three times before I went to bed.

"Oh, Len, not again!" I heard my mother say as I made my way up the stairs.

The next morning I awoke very early to find my father asleep at the kitchen table, Duke curled at his feet.

During the years of my boyhood, Duke and I explored the woods along Gwyn Oak stream, wandered the edges of the golf course. In the summers I climbed a maple tree where I would read for hours, supported in its branches, the breeze rippling through the leaves around me. Duke stretched out in the shade underneath, glanced up now and then, and waited for me to climb down. But he loved my father the most. When he heard his car coming—blocks away—he'd bark and wag his tail. On Sundays when my father worked in his rose garden, the collie stayed by his side. My father spent hours combing Duke's thick golden coat, his pure white chest. Duke sat patiently, whined only when the comb pulled too hard at a matted knot, and then, as if to make up for his ingratitude, licked my father's hand.

Duke lived for fourteen years. In the end, his kidneys failed and he limped badly from arthritis in his hips. He could no longer scramble up and down the basement steps. My father bundled this eighty-pound animal into his arms every morning and carried him up the stairs, placed him on soft bedding on the back lawn in the sun. He carried him down into the cellar each night. This went on for a few weeks, and then Duke stopped eating. One morning my father called the Humane Society and they sent a truck around. My father handed the man a twenty.

"Be gentle with him, please," he said.

My father didn't know they were going to gas Duke in the back of the truck right there in the driveway. By the time he realized what was happening, it was too late. He never got over it.

He called me at Bucknell to tell me the sad news.

"I had to put Duke down today, Jerry-boy. He was really suffering. There was nothing more I could do . . ." That was all he could say and he hung up the phone.

Several years into my practice I walked into my exam room to find one of my mentors from residency training, Dr. Sean McHenry, sitting in the chair next to my desk reading a mystery novel. He loved mysteries; he used to talk about writing a series himself when he retired.

Dr. McHenry was a nephrologist, a specialist in kidney disease, a renowned academician. During my residency he taught me the physiology of fluid and electrolyte disorders, the complex interplay of ions and hormones and cellular membranes that, in health, keep our body chemistry balanced despite what we ingest every day—and in disease, get us very quickly into serious trouble.

He was a rotund, balding man who always had a lit cigar in his mouth. The residents rotating through his service couldn't help but notice that his fingers were distinctly clubbed, like that patient I had seen during my first year of medical school. Surely, I remember thinking back then, Dr. McHenry had noticed this potentially significant medical finding at the ends of his own fingers.

"I'm honored to see you, Dr. McHenry," I said. "I hope you're just here for a checkup."

"I've been having trouble with my right thumb," he said. "It keeps twitching." Dr. McHenry was never one for small talk. He handed me an X-ray jacket containing a front and side view of his chest. "These were read as normal over at the med school," he said.

I put the films up on the view box. I stopped breathing. I saw several nodules scattered throughout both lungs. They were faint, but they were there.

"Did you look at these films?" I asked.

"What do you suggest we do?" he said.

Tests revealed that Dr. McHenry had cancer of the lung that had spread to his liver, bones, and brain. The focal motor seizures of his thumb soon progressed to his hand and arm and eventually to his whole body; a metastatic growth in the motor cortex of his left cerebral hemisphere was the culprit. He endured brain irradiation and toxic chemotherapy. He got worse and worse over the next few months, requiring anti-convulsants and pain pills. His only distraction was reading, and now he couldn't concentrate on the pages before him. "I guess I'll never write that mystery," he said one day near the end.

Soon after that I was called to the emergency room to see him. His face was gray, his lips deep blue. He groaned in pain with each breath. His respirations came in shallow, rapid gasps. His blood oxygen level measured dangerously low even on a mask with the gas fully flowing. His chest X-ray showed his enlarging tumors but nothing else—such as pneumonia—that I could potentially treat and ameliorate, for a while longer anyway.

"Dr. McHenry," I said, my mouth to his ear. The whooshing of the oxygen around his face and the general commotion in the ER made it hard for him to hear. He was soaked in sweat, his body straining with the tremendous effort to breathe; all the muscles in his neck and abdomen were working desperately to move air in and out of his lungs.

"I think you've had a pulmonary embolism," I said. "I'm going to intubate you right now and put you on a respirator." The ER nurse was standing just outside the curtained cubicle, the crash cart by her side, a laryngoscope and endotracheal tube at the ready.

"No." Dr, McHenry reached for my hand. "I'm dying," he said in short, breathless gasps. "I'm not afraid. I just can't stand this pain. Please . . ."

For a few seconds that seemed much longer, I could only squeeze his hand and look into his contorted face. I knew what I had to do but had trouble making my mouth form the words.

"Give me a syringe of morphine," I called to the nurse.

My mission, my first responsibility, is to relieve my patient's pain. Yet I knew that in relieving Dr. McHenry's pain with morphine I was going to depress his drive to breathe, and that without a ventilator, which he had just refused, he would die. Dr. McHenry, of course, knew this as well. This is the ethical dilemma of the "double-effect." I could relieve his pain, but I would shorten his life, even if only by the few minutes he could live without a respirator.

I took the syringe from the nurse and I began to push the drug through his IV tubing with my own hands.

"Good-bye, Dr. McHenry," I said.

"Thank you," he said, and soon his chest settled for the last time.

When his wife finally burst through the doors of the ER and we saw each other, I broke down; I told her what had happened and what I had done.

Mrs. McHenry, wiser than I, a woman who loved her husband,

suffered beside him as his illness progressed, and understood only too well what lay ahead had he continued to live with his cancer, took me in her arms.

"Thank you for taking such good care of him," she said.

That night my old mentor taught me one final lesson, perhaps the most important one ever. I hope I will always remember it, that I will be brave enough when it is my time to choose.

FOURTEEN

When my parents left Baltimore, my father cleaned out the basement on Green Meadow Parkway, our home after we had moved from Forest Park. He was maniacal about it. On the curb he piled box upon box: my brother's and my boyhood toys, my chemistry cabinet, my brother's erector set, our electric trains, my college notebooks, the few business supplies salvaged from the old pawnshop, his photographic equipment, our Ping-Pong table, net, balls and paddles, seldom-used kitchen utensils. He was intent on throwing out the clutter, anything superfluous that would remind him of his old life.

My father abandoned the city of his birth and youth and middle years; he left his three siblings who were still alive at that time. But two items from our basement escaped the trash heap: the wooden easel he had had since his youth and which had gathered dust my entire life, and an oil painting completed when he was only sixteen, a portrait of a neighbor's gardener: a black man in a brown suit, his white shirt buttoned all the way to the top.

As soon as he moved into his San Antonio home, my father un-
folded his easel in a corner of the garage, wired up bright fluorescent
lighting, and went searching for paints and brushes and canvas. At the
local library he spent hours studying art books. And then came the
paintings: my daughters at every age, the children of friends and rel-
atives, his mother and his siblings modeled from old photographs,
scenes of the Texas hill country, shrimp boats on the coast, the River-
walk, impressionistic renditions of birds, rose bushes, irises, and hy-
drangeas from his garden. Sometimes he painted all night long. He
experimented with pastels and watercolors and acrylics, painted on
wood and glass, mixed sand and other materials into his paints, spread
the colors with palette knives and rags, broom straw and sticks. He
built his own frames. His shoes were always covered in paint; the
garage floor around his workspace looked like a Jackson Pollock.

I hung many of his finished works in my medical office. The
exhibit constantly morphed. My patients raved about his paintings.
One man, a serious artist and museum patron, wanted to put on a show
of my father's oils in his own private gallery. My father wouldn't consider it. "I don't have the faintest idea what I'm doing," he said. "I'm
just a piker." He never sold a single painting; nor did he ever try.

What might his life have been had he attended art school, had he
not spent his best years in the pawnshop?

"Did you know that my maiden name is Winokur?" the poet Maxine Kumin asked me when we met at the Vermont Studio Center in
1994. She was then almost seventy, but her athletic frame, bright
eyes, and broad smile made her seem years younger. "We spell it
with an 'o,'" she said, "but you know those immigration officers on
Ellis Island—it was all phonetic."

I had come to Vermont—at the age of forty-seven—to sit around
a table with a few other "wannabe" poets as she critiqued our work
and we tried to learn something more of this art, her art. I'd been
reading her poetry for years, admired her connection to the natural

world. I left my patients and my family to make this journey, to what end I wasn't certain. I had watched my father find some measure of redemption through his art, rediscovered late in life. I didn't know if poetry could do the same for me, but at least no one would die if I mixed my metaphors.

That was the beginning of a friendship between Maxine and me. Over the last decade my wife Lee and I have become close friends with Maxine and her husband, Victor. We've visited PoBiz Farm, the Kumins' home in New Hampshire, walked the forest paths and the pastures—including the aptly named Elysian Field—strolled the riding ring while Maxine worked out with her horses, swum naked in the pond (well, Lee did), and plucked fresh vegetables from Maxine's bountiful garden. I have mucked out the stalls and helped Victor clear the drain under the paddock as I crouched up to my shoulders in weeds and manure.

The Kumins have stayed with us at our ranch in Texas, as well. Victor, with his practical engineer's mind, helped us prioritize all the work we needed to do when Lee and I first bought our rundown place in the hill country, less than an hour from the hustle and bustle of San Antonio. I remember how intent Victor was: To this day, remnants of orange surveyor tape flutter from the critical areas he marked for us: plumbing connections, irrigation heads, electrical junction boxes.

After Maxine met my father, she told me he reminded her of her favorite brother, dead years ago from Lou Gehrig's disease, a wasting neurodegenerative process that took him, muscle by muscle, away from her. She understood my father's yearning to find time and space for his artistic life and she complimented him on his work. "I think she really likes my paintings," he said to me again and again after one of her visits.

Perhaps there is shared blood between Maxine Kumin and me. I have been the surrogate son for so many older folks that it has been a joy to find a set of surrogate parents, though this has not been without responsibility.

On July 21, 1998, I received an e-mail from Victor. Maxine had just broken her neck during a carriage-driving competition. She was on a respirator, her situation dire. I did a quick calculation in my head: She was seventy-three years old, Victor five years her senior. But these were not the old old I was accustomed to in my own family; not the ones I usually see in my practice. They were more active than many half their ages: riding horses, swimming in the pond, mucking out stalls, weeding the garden. Still, I know, when anyone Maxine's age has a severe setback, the dominoes begin to fall.

I called Victor and I learned more details: Maxine had a punctured lung, multiple rib fractures, internal bleeding, contusions of her liver and kidney, and a loss of neurological function in her arms and legs. I remembered Maxine's medical history: breast cancer, coronary artery disease, and a longstanding inflammatory muscle condition requiring cortisone therapy. And now this. My doctor's head was spinning; I didn't see how she could possibly survive. If she did, she would be in a wheelchair the rest of her days. And then I thought: No. Not Maxine. She will find a way out of that.

She tells the story of this ordeal in her book, *Inside the Halo and Beyond: The Anatomy of a Recovery*. She spends months in a "halo cast," a birdcage-like contraption, worn over her head and supported on her torso, that holds her fractured neck in proper alignment via screws drilled into her skull. She endures great pain, months of physical therapy, and overcomes depression. By reaching deep inside—to a wellspring of poems committed to memory—she finds the strength to survive. And always her family is steadfast. Her daughter, Judith, takes dictation as Maxine recounts the daily trials for her memoir in progress.

But even Maxine—stalwart and determined as she is—draws a line in the sand. In late October 1998, it appears that she might need surgery to stabilize her cervical spine. She is panicked at the possibility that she might wake up unable to move her arms and legs, that this paralysis might be permanent. She has worked so hard these last months to regain some strength and mobility in her limbs.

Maxine e-mails me. She wants my assurance that if, as a result of this surgery, she awakens a quadriplegic, I will agree to come and—in her words—"put her down."

"I am not depressed and I am not insane," she writes. "I have made my wishes very clear to all the family, but I think they are too emotionally involved to take action. So, don't lecture me; just E-mail me one word, *Yes* or *No*." In her book she says that I "fired back my answer."* But she did not know how much I agonized over it.

"*Put her down*"—a neutral term, shorn of emotion. But for me to put her down meant murdering her, an illegal act, a felony, one for which I might rot in jail. How could I possibly answer her in any way but "No"?

Instead I said "Yes." I am a pragmatist, an advocate in for the long haul. I knew Maxine was asking for reassurance, for her worst fears to be acknowledged, for her suffering to be understood.

At the time I had no doubt that she would have forgiven me had I not been able to follow through. I was gambling—I was praying—that my service in this regard would not be needed, or that when the time came she would choose to go on with whatever strength and will and inner fire she could muster, as she has always done and continues to do to this day. But she needed to hear from me in the affirmative at that panicked moment in her life, and I knew it.

She knew full well what she had asked of me. In her memoir she writes: "I carry my brother's story around with me like a very heavy knapsack. First he lost the use of his legs, then his arms, then his ability to speak, and finally even his fingers turned to stone. I am trying to make provisions for my own exit just as he did. But probably just as he could not rely on me, I will not be able to rely even on my faithful friend of the one-word E-mail."

Fortunately for Maxine and her family, for all of us, she survived that ordeal in 1998. Her neck finally fused on its own. She has persevered. Since then, she has published four more books. At age eighty-one—and after double hip replacements—she is again riding her horse. Maxine and Victor are stellar examples of how a physically vigorous and intellectually stimulating old age can help us approach our biologically determined maximum life spans.

But what if things had not turned out so well, if her worst fears had been realized?

I think back to that night in the ER with my old mentor, Dr. McHenry. He was a competent patient with an incurable disease and he was drawing his last few breaths no matter what I did. I gave him enough morphine to ease his pain; the drug suppressed his respirations and he died in a few minutes instead of ten or twenty spent in great distress.

But from this point on in the ethical debate over end-of-life issues, we are on a very slippery slope.

What about the patient with cancer whose pain is mostly relieved by the excellent palliative care available today, someone who could perhaps live a few more months, but the existential angst, the breakthrough episodes of pain, and the physical deterioration are just too much, and she asks her physician for his assistance in dying? Dr. Timothy Quill wrote about just such a patient, "Diane," in a landmark article published in the *New England Journal of Medicine*. He gave her a prescription for barbiturates, for "both sleep and suicide." Diane took them all and Dr. Quill was charged with murder. A grand jury refused to indict him.

It is exactly this scenario that the Oregon Death With Dignity Act—passed in two separate referenda by the people of that state—was designed to address. Physician assisted suicide (PAS) is legal in Oregon if the patient requesting it is clearly competent and dying of a terminal disease with less than six months to live. There must be a fifteen-day waiting period and the physician may only prescribe the fatal dose, not administer it. The Act has been invoked in relatively few cases, but it has been used.

There have been some valid arguments made against PAS: concerns that palliative care is not being adequately utilized; that some patients may still be depressed (there is no requirement for a psychiatric evaluation in Oregon's law); that financial issues—especially in these days of limited resources and managed care—might prevail over ethical ones.

Some ethicists argue that once an initial step like PAS is in place, something sinister in human nature will take over; that once we as a society change our laws and practices even in a small way, our ability to reason and extrapolate will be extended to more and more situations.

The philosopher Peter Singer argues that PAS in response to a competent patient's request is perfectly defensible. In fact, Singer believes that some people—children with severe disabilities, for example— would have been better off not being born, that their lives are somehow less well-lived.

In her book, *Too Late to Die Young,* Harriet McBryde Johnson, a disability rights attorney who is herself confined to a wheelchair, counters Singer with a simple but powerful observation: "(T)he presence or absence of a disability doesn't predict the quality of life." What makes the lives of so many disabled people miserable, she argues, why some of them ask to be "put down," is that society has failed them; that pervasive prejudice against the disabled prevents us from taking proper care of them in the first place.

As a geriatrician working in America today, when the number of folks between sixty-five and seventy-four will double in the next forty-five years, the number between seventy-five and eighty-four will more than double, and those over eighty-five will *quadruple* to eighteen million—I worry that our elderly are on track to become "the other." In the category of the oldest old, half will be demented and only one out of twenty will be fully mobile. Faced with this burden—on our caregivers and families, on our personal finances, on our nation's resources—how far will our society be willing to slide down that slippery slope?

My father and I are sitting together on my parents' back patio. It's early evening, summer; a slight breeze has come up out of the southeast. It is quiet, the only sound a neighbor's dog barking a few houses down. My father turns to me and says, "Do you remember Duke?"

"Of course, Dad. He was a great dog, wasn't he?"

"I didn't think you were around then."

"Sure, I was. I remember the night we brought him home, that terrible snowstorm . . ."

"I must have been crazy," he says.

"You were just trying to be a good father."

"I didn't know they were going to kill him right there in the backyard. I thought they would take him away somewhere . . ."

"Dad, Duke was old and sick and in a lot of pain."

"I used to carry him up and down the cellar steps every day there for a while . . . I couldn't do it anymore."

"You did the best you could."

"I just wish they wouldn't have killed him right there in the backyard. Gassed him, like the damn Nazis . . ."

I watch my father's face, see the tears begin to well. I put my hand on his arm.

"Dad, Duke was dying."

"I know." He takes out his handkerchief and blows his nose. "Let that be a lesson to you," he says.

He surprises me with this statement. When I was a boy, this line always preceded a pronouncement of his hard-earned wisdom. What is my father thinking now? Is he telling me to put him down when the time comes? That he doesn't want to suffer and linger?

"Dad, what do you mean? What sort of 'lesson'? Tell me . . ."

"I don't want to talk about it," he says.

FIFTEEN

Six years ago my mother called me late one night. Her voice trembled on the other end of the line.

"Your father is pacing back and forth. He keeps opening the door. 'I need fresh air . . . I can't breathe . . .' he's saying. I don't know what to do . . ."

"I'm coming over," I said.

I had been waiting for my father to have more heart trouble. Since his heart attack fifteen years before, his cardiac function had been poor, but with medications he'd done reasonably well. Until tonight.

I took one look at him—his pallor and gray-blue lips, his rapid, shallow breathing, his distended neck veins—and knew that his lungs were filling up with fluid as a result of a failing heart.

"Dad, you've got to go into the hospital for a few days, okay?" I knew he didn't want to go. I understood what an ordeal this was likely to be.

"Whatever you say," he said. His refusal to argue made me worry all the more.

I called Dr. Galan. "I'm bringing my father into the ER. He's in heart failure," I said.

"I'll be there," he said.

There is nothing more reassuring to a family in an emergency than to hear their doctor say these words.

My father was admitted to the same hospital in which I have made rounds almost every day of my life for the last three decades. I know many of the nurses and therapists by first name. The CEO is my friend and patient. Dr. John Galan, my father's physician, is smart, well trained, and compassionate. I was confident that my father would receive the best medical care available in America today; yet I would not leave him alone in his hospital room.

Acute hospitalizations are the most dangerous times for the elderly. Even if they have never before manifested any signs of confusion or disorientation, it is in the hospital, in a strange and threatening environment, under the influence of anesthetics, pain pills, anti-emetics, and soporifics, that the elderly—competent or not—meet their match. Add to this the iatrogenic mishaps (the "normally expected" side effects and complications of standard medical procedures and therapies) and human errors multiplying in our modern hospitals like germs in a petri dish (mistakes in drug dosing or the right medication given to the wrong patient, to name just two), and it is a miracle any elderly patient gets out of the hospital unscathed.

I stayed with my father every night, slept in the reclining chair by his bed. I got up when he did, ran interference with bed rails, side tables, and IV poles, guarded his every move to the bathroom, inspected every medication that was handed to him, every fluid-filled bag plugged into his arm. I was not afraid to question the nurse or call his physician. Nevertheless, each day my father descended deeper and deeper into paranoid confusion.

"Why am I locked up in here?" he said. "Get me out, Jerry-boy. Take me home. Please!"

He couldn't rest; he was intermittently unsure of who I was. At first I could calm him with my voice, talking about the old days, reminding him of our fishing trips on the Chesapeake, the birds we have seen together. Then he needed the physical reassurance of my hand on his arm or shoulder. Finally, so that he could sleep, I got in the bed with him and held him, comforting him as he once, in a long-ago life, comforted me.

My father had developed delirium, an increasingly common and dangerous condition that stalks our elderly in our modern hospitals today. Take large numbers of frail folks, people with multiple underlying medical problems on long lists of drugs, who are barely holding on in their own home environments, and it is just a matter of time before many will—in the hospital—become confused, paranoid, belligerent, and a danger to themselves as well as their caregivers. The delirium itself can be a fatal complication of a hospital stay; once the few triggering causes (such as drugs, infections, and body chemistry imbalances) are investigated and corrected, the delirium may remain even after discharge. This is particularly true for our loved ones who already manifest a degree of dementia, recognized or not.

After four days and nights I knew I had to get my father out of the hospital.

"Your dad's heart failure is better," Dr. Galan said to me. "But he's still more confused than he was when he came in. And deconditioned. Why don't we put him in the SNU for a bit?"

At that time I was the medical director of the Skilled Nursing Unit (SNU). After all, Dr. Galan rightly believed, my father could expect good care there.

When an attending physician feels his patient no longer needs the services of the acute hospital setting but is still not ready to return home, the SNU may be a good alternative. Sometimes it is obvious what we have to do when a patient comes to the SNU: finish out a course of intravenous antibiotics in a patient with an infected wound, provide a few more days of rehab to a competent elder who has just undergone a hip replacement; but more and more, as our patients grow older and frailer, the attending physician requests a transfer to the SNU because she doesn't know what to do next.

Each week I attended the SNU Team Care Conference. Team care is at the heart of modern geriatric medicine.

Around the table sit a registered nurse, a geriatric nurse specialist, pharmacist, social worker, activity coordinator, physical, occupational, speech, and respiratory therapists, licensed vocational nurses (LVNs) who provide most of the daily nursing care, a dietician, and myself.

"What progress has Mr. Jones made with his physical therapy this past week?" I will ask.

"Mrs. Smith has developed diarrhea. She was recently placed on an antibiotic for a urinary infection. Should we look into this?" the RN might ask me.

"I haven't been able to get in touch with anyone in Mr. White's family at all yet," the social worker will say. "There's nowhere for him to go."

"And he's still losing weight," the dietician will add.

Our main goal at this weekly meeting is to answer one major question: What are we going to do with this patient? Where can we safely send him—given all the exigencies of his medical, social, and financial circumstances—and expect him to maintain his highest level of function, his remaining dignity? Very often, we don't know.

"I think perhaps we should transfer your father to our Skilled Nursing Unit for some rehabilitation," the doctor says. I say it all the time. You are uncertain what this means except that you don't have to take Dad home just yet. You are temporarily grateful. The doctor has postponed answering the "What are we going to do with Dad?" question for a while longer. Every Medicare patient has coverage for one hundred lifetime SNU days *if* the criteria outlined in the regulations are met, but beyond the first week or two it's often difficult to meet these criteria—*not* because the patient is well enough to live independently but because he is, in the words of the regulators, "no longer making progress." He is caught in the downward spiral of old age, disability, and dementia.

So after your dad has his week or two in the SNU and you have returned to the old environs you thought you'd left behind forever, you realize finally that your father is totally incapable of negotiating the real world. You've been visiting a few times a year, calling once or twice a week. He talks about the weather and asks about your kids. His dementia has been coming on for years, but you were ignorant of or chose to ignore the more subtle signs: the superficiality of your conversations, the occasional outburst, the gradual withdrawal from community and friends, the unkempt appearance, the messy home. And now he is in the SNU still covered by Medicare at least for the next week or two and you don't have a clue what to do with him after that.

Perhaps you'll join the ranks of unpaid American family caregivers who supply the bulk of long-term care for their loved ones. Today that's fifty million volunteer caregivers, more than one quarter of all adults. Of course, spouses constitute the largest group of these; daughters are next, contributing 20 percent of this care to their elderly parents or their in-laws. Sons do not, in general, do their part—only 6 percent of them are involved in the long-term care of our elderly. The average length of time each of us may be involved in the care of our elderly parents is eight years, although one third of folks may spend ten years or more in this caregiving role.

What else can I do with my father now? What options exist for "long-term care"? In the last decade or so the long-term care industry has begun an evolution from a hospital model to a hotel or concierge model. Perhaps this was done to avoid the heavy regulatory oversight imposed on the traditional nursing-home business and create another niche—the assisted-living industry—which was, in the beginning, almost totally unregulated.

The big hotel corporations got into long-term care. Hotel chains knew all about amenities: nice lobbies, pools, landscaped grounds, appealing meals. Unfortunately they knew little or nothing about the elderly who, to no one's surprise, "aged-in-place," that is, became increasingly frail and demented as they lived on in their well-appointed rooms. No one was around to recognize there was a problem until the old folks started breaking hips, getting lost, forgetting to take their medications.

Many lawsuits later, the assisted-living industry is now coming under more scrutiny; a number of states are adopting regulations requiring on-site nursing and medical support, pharmacy support, and—in the most enlightened places—certified long-term-care medical directors (mandated decades ago in custodial nursing homes) to oversee the care. Not surprisingly, because of this heightened oversight, the hotel industry is now getting out of the assisted-living business. Undoubtedly some new entity will sidle in to take over the business of delivering "quality care" to our seniors.

So what is the definition of "quality care" for our loved ones in institutional settings? Given the multiplicity of medical conditions that plague our elderly, the complexity of their management needs, their increasing frailty—can we even begin to define what constitutes "quality care" for the two million people admitted to the seventeen thousand nursing homes in America each year? Experts are trying to come up with parameters to define quality, but the task is fraught with difficulties. One panel of geriatricians wrestling with "quality indicators" (QIs)—steps of care associated with better outcomes—concluded that only six out of twenty-two such QIs were "valid but of questionable feasibility to implement considering the resources available in an average community nursing home trying to provide quality care."

"Quality care" probably means different things to medical professionals than it does to patients and their families. The nursing home may do a splendid job, for example, in its "care processes" to manage heart failure in a given patient. But if it takes the nurse a half hour to answer the call bell or an hour to change the patient's bedding after an accident, well, neither the patient nor his family will be very happy with the care rendered, no matter how high the home scores on "quality indicators."

Another example illustrates just how hard it is to measure quality in long-term care: pressure ulcer development in our institutionally housed elders. These areas of skin breakdown over bony prominences have long been considered markers for "poor" care by patients and their families, government regulators, and, of course, malpractice plaintiff attorneys. And it seems obvious, doesn't it? The occurrence of a pressure sore means that someone wasn't doing his job—not turning the patient enough, not protecting the skin, not ensuring adequate nutrition, and on and on. There is always plenty of blame, and the nursing home record—an imperfect document always—is paraded in front of the jury as damning evidence of "poor quality care."

The truth is so much more complex than this. Many studies have shown that there is "no link between documentation of a quality indicator and incidence of pressure ulcers . . . no difference in direct clinical observation of processes of care between nursing facilities with low and high pressure ulcer incidence." Two experts concluded that "despite the development of clinical guidelines, new strategies for prevention interventions, and considerable attention paid to reducing the incidence of pressure ulcers, the long-term effect of prevention strategies remains problematic. No change in pressure ulcer prevalence (in a nationally derived sample of long-term nursing home residents) has been observed since . . . 1987."

Pressure ulcers, then, are not necessarily markers for poor nursing-home care, but rather for something as yet incompletely understood about the biological nature of these sores and the yet-to-be-discovered best ways to prevent and ultimately heal them. One thing is clear: They have not and will not be cured by multi-million-dollar judgments against doctors and nursing homes.

Of course we will need excellent examples of institutionally based long-term care, and these models will need to be monitored and refined over time. But our aging society needs much more new thinking about this subject. We must have nothing less than a total transformation.

Many of my boomer brethren believe that technology will save us. They've grown up on *Star Trek*, made money in high tech; they carry all the latest electronic gadgets, worship at the feet of futurist gurus like Ray Kurzweil, who takes hundreds of pills daily to "re-program" his body chemistry in order to live out his maximal biological life span—one hundred to one hundred twenty years or so. By then, he assures us, we will be able to download our "wet" brains into "dry" cyborgian creations and "live" forever.

Yes, technology is advancing; we've heard the Silicone Valley mantra—"smaller, faster, cheaper"—over and over. This merging of engineering, biology, genetics, and physics does have the potential to benefit mankind. Of course, the opposite may happen, technology may make us less human, may reduce us to mechanical creatures living in virtual realities, bereft of our squishy wet bodies that are so prone to oxidation and rust, to non-upgradable aging.

Technology without wisdom is like a runaway horse. It may take us very quickly to somewhere we don't want to go. Our elderly need *people*—friends, family members, and health-care workers who understand and value them as individuals—all of them crucial to providing quality care to our aging loved ones. We must work to-gether to decide when to embrace the latest technological advance and when to turn away.

What about the price tag for all this care? There may be govern-mental safety nets—as there are now with state Medicaid programs—but unless there is radical new thinking about how we will care for our parents and then ourselves, we are all going to be in for a very rude awakening.

What is state-of-the-art when it comes to long-term care for our el-derly? For that matter, can we even agree on what the goals of long-term care should be? Many of us—but not all—believe that "quality of life" is more important than "length of life."

What is "quality of life" when one is demented? When the families of my chronically ill and cognitively impaired patients come to me for advice, when they are ready to make the move into long-term custodial care, I tell them to take a deep breath. Many have already done some research and investigated a few facilities. I explain how important it is for the facility to be close to family and friends. I tell them not to be swayed by how new or swanky the building, grounds, and lobby appear. Cosmetics bear little correlation to the care delivered. Some families are put off by foul odors. Given the resident population, the "smell test" may not be a fair assessment of quality.

I tell them to talk to the other families, look into the faces of the residents, observe how they are dressed and cared for. Ask about the length of time staff members—especially the aides—have worked there. Long employment is a sign that the staff is satisfied with the institution.

I advise my families to visit the facility more than once, at different times of the day, when the residents are being given their daily care, when they are being fed or taken to the dining room. Make sure there are adequate dietary and physical therapy services, that staff responsible for activity planning and spiritual well-being are available.

And remember—no decision is irreversible. If things are not going well, if the facility is not meeting your expectations, sit down with the administrator and director of nursing. Outline your concerns. If nothing changes, don't be afraid to move on.

For those in my generation, there are some heartening developments in this growing arena of retirement and long-term-care options.

Homesharing is one of these concepts. Seniors who need help with the activities of daily living open their doors—through a matching system—to a younger person or couple, who will, in exchange for a place to live, assist the elder with these tasks. There are even organizations that match elders to elders, where one's strength is in the area of another's weakness.

Here's another interesting idea: Naturally Occurring Retirement

Communities (NORCs) are popping up all over the country. In Manhattan, for example, there's a hundred-unit apartment building for aging "women in the arts." Female artists can age in place together, "living and working until the end of life." There are common areas for dining, lectures, readings, and art exhibitions. In Virginia, residents grow grapes, produce their own vintage wines, and oversee their own dinner menus. In New Mexico, a project based on the Buddhist principles of interconnectedness and respect for the earth will house people who have devoted their lives to social activism and spiritual development. They plan a meditation hall, health-care unit, and a hospice.

Beacon Hill Village in Boston is a "non-profit organization created by and for local residents determined to grow old in familiar surroundings," which is to say, of course, their own homes. This organization provides transportation to and from medical care, home-delivered meals from favorite restaurants, emergency response at the ready, and people stopping by just to check. The group was formed because the individuals involved "were unwilling to be herded into cookie-cutter senior housing and told what to do by social workers half their age."

Nationwide there are now more than one hundred communities similar to Beacon Hill—"villages" as some call themselves—that have arisen in response to this one certain and growing realization: Unless enthusiastic and robust individuals begin to take the initiative to plan for and implement self-empowering strategies for their aged years, there will be no one to do it for them. Witness the proposed "aging in place" experiments authorized but never funded in the 2006 Older American Act.

At the other end of the spectrum, in Texas, an RV park lies deep in the piney woods north of Houston. Here, for less than the cost of an apartment, residents live in their own RVs and receive "virtually all the care offered by assisted living—meals, housecleaning, laundry, transportation, activities, and nursing care."

For those who want to continue learning as long as they can,

University Living in Ann Arbor and Independence Grove at Hillsdale College, both in Michigan, are affiliations between an elder living environment and a university, places where aging men and women can take classes and live alongside college students.

These examples—experiments, really—in retirement and senior living are all about people taking control of their own lives, making decisions about their elder years while they still can. In most of these NORCs the residents have made arrangements for health-care professionals to live on the premises and for doctors to visit regularly. These people want to control how and where they die, not just where they live. They are not being passive in the face of old age and death. They discuss, they plan, they implement.

When the time came for me to make a decision for my father during his last hospital stay, I took him home. Dr. Galan understood why I chose this route: I knew that given my father's confusion and paranoia, a transfer to yet another hospital unit would only have added to his agitation; more medications would have been required to subdue the delirium demons. For my father, the Skilled Nursing Unit would have been only another stop on the way to long-term custodial nursing-home care.

So I brought my father home. I arranged for a home health agency to come to my parents' house, to give my father physical therapy and help with bathing and dressing and grooming. I went to the pharmacy and filled the eight prescriptions Dr. Galan wrote out for him. When I realized that even with a magnifying lens my mother could no longer read the labels on the bottles, I went back again to buy the blue plastic container divided into daily dosing compartments.

The Medicare coverage for the home health agency ran out almost as soon as it had begun. Between my brother and me, one of us is there almost every day. We have been fortunate to find a dedicated home-care worker, Yolanda, who helps my father shave and shower and dress each morning. She helps my mother with shopping and cooking, the laundry, and keeping the house straight.

On the supplemental nutritional liquid feedings my brother brings to the house by the case, my father has put on a few pounds. I keep his medicines stocked and I fiddle with the doses now and then—a tad extra diuretic when l see he is more short of breath, a tiny dose of an antipsychotic if he becomes more agitated. We take him to Dr. Galan regularly for follow-up exams and lab tests. And still, every week he gets worse, harder to deal with, more bizarre.

For most of last week he hollered at my mother when she tried to help him change his pants because he had wet himself. "You're my sister! You're not supposed to see me naked!" he screamed. He can no longer find his way from the living room to his bedroom in their small one-story home.

One day you may get a call. Your father is confused and was found wandering the streets many blocks from his home. Or your mother has had a stroke and is now in an intensive care unit. Or he broke his hip after he fell off a ladder. The house is a mess, the fire department says, because she left the toaster oven on, a loaf of bread in a plastic bag sitting on top of it. And this brings you back to your old hometown, takes you away from your family, your job. Your spouse is now chief cook and bottle washer, full-time carpool person. Your boss is irritated, but you've got the Family Medical Leave Act on your side, at least for a while.

You spend day after day in a cramped hospital room; you exercise by wiping the floor so your father doesn't slip in his own urine. Your mother isn't exactly sure who you are, but she puts on a good front when the doctor comes by; he is planning to send her home at the end of the week. "Is she really okay to go home?" you ask. You know the answer; but if *she* can go home maybe *you* can go home and pick up your busy life where you dropped it a week or a month ago. "Dad can handle Mom," you tell yourself. Or maybe, "Aunt Greta will be there to lend a hand" or "My brother only lives a two-hour drive away. It's about time he stepped up to the plate . . ."

Stop deluding yourself. It's time to have some tough discussions—sisters, brothers, Mom and Dad. It's time to make plans.

SIXTEEN

In early November 2005 I pull into my parents' driveway. A few nights before the temperature had dropped into the upper thirties as the first norther of the season blew through town, but today the high is seventy-five and the cloudless sky is as blue as the iris of a newborn. There is a flock of cedar waxwings—early for this time of year—gorging themselves on pyracantha berries. My father planted the bushes around his house years ago just to attract these winter visitors.

I have finished up with my patients a bit early, and since this is flu shot season I have brought a pre-loaded syringe of vaccine for my father. I will administer it myself, something I have done the last few years to save my father an extra trip into the doctor's office. In his weakened condition, with the progressive decline in his ability to walk, getting him out of the house is now a major logistical feat.

I am still sitting in my car in the driveway. There is a letter on the seat beside me that I fished out of my mail pile just before I left the office. The envelope has no return address, is postmarked from another state, and the letter itself is unsigned. I had read the first few lines, then stuffed it back into the envelope and carried it out to my car intending to finish it later. I pick it up again. It begins:

> *Re: "What Are We Going to Do with Dad"*
> *Dear Dr. Winakur:*
>
> *I was very disappointed in your article above, which appeared in the newspaper. How could you possibly torture your own father and prolong his dying like you are doing??? What kind of fiend are you????*

This was as far as I'd gotten when I opened the letter. Apparently my essay which first appeared in *Health Affairs* and then in the *Washington Post* had now been reprinted in another local newspaper. I force myself to continue.

> *Your father's major problem is medicarditis. If he and his family, meaning you, had to pay for his dying directly, rather than palming it off onto working families with children via medicare, your father would have died a natural death three years ago with his CHF. I guarantee it . . .*

I sense that this author is not some ignorant deranged reactionary—"CHF" is a commonly used medical abbreviation for congestive heart failure. I feel an urge to tear up the page and toss it into the garbage, but I keep reading.

> *Now I realize that the medical-industrial complex uses demented old people as cash cows and ATM machines all the time, but to do that to your own father???? Why???? How terribly cruel you are! Don't you remember when we were all in residency and wanted to tattoo "DNR" (Do Not Resuscitate) onto our own chests?? There was a reason for that, we knew back then the care was futile . . .*

Well, now is the time to do that favor for your own father . . . And tattoo "Do Not Call 911" onto his chest, too, while you're about it . . .

My fear is confirmed. This person—too cowardly to sign his name—is a physician. He goes on:

What are we going to do with Dad? The answer is simple . . . We are going to let God be God. We are going to let nature take its course. If he dies, he dies. If he lives, he lives. . . . No flu shots, no calling 911, no antibiotics, no trips to the hospital . . . They're better off dead . . . Death is inevitable for all of us . . . One can die quick. Or one can die slowly, tortured by a son like you . . .

I fold the letter back into its envelope and pick up the syringe of flu vaccine. The vaccine costs ten dollars a dose from the manufacturer, which is just about what Medicare reimburses us for each shot we administer at the time of a patient's office visit. There is only one reason a group practice like mine goes through this each year: because we believe it is the right thing to do for our geriatric patients. Here is what is entailed: We must order the vaccine, pay for it—including any unused doses—store it, sort it, draw it up into syringes (which we supply at our own expense), schedule and debrief each patient, get them to sign special forms, administer each shot, record each vaccination in each medical record, assume the liability for each untoward reaction, generate an electronic insurance claim to Medicare, and wait months to get paid. Geriatricians have always stood at the wrong orifice of the Medicare "cash cow" to which my so-called colleague refers.

I am remembering the nightmare of my father's last hospital stay as I get out of the car and walk to my parents' front door. Two white-wing doves coo and then flush from the pecan tree. I let myself in. As usual, it is dark inside. My parents don't believe in sunlight. My mother worries it will fade her forty-year-old sofa while at the same time she bemoans the fact that her plants always die. My father insists the curtains remain closed so no one can peer in.

My mother is asleep in the recliner, in front of the blaring television. Whenever I visit, my first move is to find the remote and mute the TV. This wakes her. I kiss her forehead. Her silver hair is all poufed up and smells like shampoo. This morning she went for her regular weekly visit to the beauty shop; my brother delivered her, and my wife picked her up and then took her to lunch, bringing her back in time for Yolanda to leave.

"Oh, you're here," my mother says.

I open the curtains. "It's a gorgeous day," I say. "I stopped by to give Dad his flu shot."

"Your father's asleep—as usual," she says.

"Well, looks to me like you're both taking a siesta."

"He's been keeping me up at night again with his wandering and raving," she says.

"Are you remembering to give him his nighttime medicine for agitation?" I ask, knowing she is always trying to cut back on it because it dulls his mental processes even further.

"I guess I'll have to start it up again," she says. "You know it makes him sleepy the next day . . ."

"Mom . . . we've been through this a hundred times . . ." I walk the short hall to my father's bedroom. He is asleep.

"Dad," I say gently. Then a bit louder, "Dad." I put my hand on his shoulder.

He opens his eyes and is frightened. He is trying to make sense of what he sees, where he is, who I am.

"Dad, it's me. Jerry. How are you feeling today?"

"Jerry-boy—is that really you?" I see in his eyes that the fear and confusion are subsiding. "You don't come around much anymore, do you?" he says.

"I come over here all the time. Why don't you let me help you up and into the living room? Mom is there. We'll visit a while . . ."

"Mom? Where is Mom? . . . I thought she was dead."

"No, Dad. Mom is your wife . . . my mother. Come, you'll see her in the living room. It's a beautiful day—maybe you'd like to sit outside. There's a flock of cedar waxwings eating your pyracantha berries . . ."

"What?" he says. "Waxwhat . . . ?"

"Waxwings, Dad. You remember—golden body, black face, crest . . ."

"I don't know what you're saying . . . I don't feel so hot. Let me go back to sleep, will you? Please!" I don't want to push him further, but maybe I can distract him.

"Okay, Dad, okay. Go back to sleep. Just one quick thing . . . let me give you your flu shot. It'll only take a second."

"My what?"

"You know, the flu shot. I give it to you every year so you won't get the flu or pneumonia. I have it right here in this syringe ready for you . . ."

"Do you know what you're doing with that?"

"Dad, I'm a doctor. Your son the doctor, remember?"

"How long have you been a doctor?"

"Over thirty years now, Dad."

"I can't believe it. Really, has it been thirty years?"

"Time flies. What do you say, Dad, how about I give you this flu shot now?"

"By all means," he says. "Thirty years, I don't believe it."

It only takes a few seconds.

"How was that?"

"I didn't feel a thing," he says.

He is now distracted and calmer, so I try again.

"Dad, why don't you let me help you into the living room and you and Mom and I will visit a bit?"

"Mom is here?" he asks.

"Yes, Dad. She's in the living room."

"Well, sure," he says. "I'd love to see Mom."

I help him find his glasses, balance him on the side of the bed, set his walker in front of him, give him a boost to his feet.

"I'm weak as a kitten," he says. He pushes his walker and I follow closely behind. "God, I feel like an old man," he says. I notice that his left leg drags a little and I wonder if perhaps he's had a mild stroke. I make a mental note to speak with Dr. Galan about this in the morning. Maybe he'll agree that my father might benefit from some physical therapy.

"There she is," he says. He has rounded the hall into the living room and he catches sight of my mother in her chair, her silver hair radiating the light now streaming in from the open window. "My beautiful wife," he says, suddenly abandoning his walker and making a lunge for the corner of the couch next to her chair.

"Dad, what are you doing? You're going to fall!"

"I want to sit down next to my beautiful wife," he says. Somehow he makes it to the sofa. He is short of breath from this very brief exertion.

"Now I'm his wife again," my mother says to me. "This morning I was his sister."

"What do you mean?" my father asks. "Of course you're my wife . . . don't you think I know my own wife? And I love you. You know I love you, don't you?"

"Yeah, I know," my mother says.

"And she loves you, too, Dad," I say.

"Of course she does," he says. "We've been married a long time, haven't we, Mom? How long have we been married?"

"Fifty-nine years," she says, her expression grim.

He turns to me. "Did you hear what she said, 'fifty-nine years'? That's a helluva of a long time, you know . . . and I've loved every minute of it. Haven't you loved every minute of it, Mom?"

"Oh, yeah. Every minute."

"What'd I tell you?" he says to me.

I don't answer him. The TV is on, muted, yet CNN manages to

blare even without the sound. Bits of information crawl across the bottom of the screen like ants at a picnic. Today it's all about the scare over avian influenza: the very real fear that a global pandemic will kill tens of millions, hundreds of millions.

I think about my anonymous colleague and his letter. There is more to his diatribe:

> *With enemies like you as a son, your father desperately needs a*
> *good friend like pneumonia to help him now in his time of need . . .*

Of course, these end-of-life care issues are complex. But the author of this letter is a doctor. Where is his empathy, his humanity? How can he presume to put himself in my place, in my father or mother's place?

I take the remote from my mother's lap and turn off the television. I sit back down in the chair and study my parents. I shouldn't get into this, but I can't help myself.

"Dad," I say, "are you happy?"

He looks at me for a few seconds, then back to my mother. Outside the window the waxwings are gorging themselves, coming and going in throngs, diving into the clusters of red berries.

"Frances, am I happy?" he asks her. My mother releases the lever on her La-Z-Boy. Her body springs to attention.

"I can't answer that for you, Leonard," she says. "You have to answer for yourself."

My father looks back at me. He wants my help. I think back to his last hospital stay, just five years ago. How helpless and confused he was then. So far I have kept my promise to him and to myself. He remains at home. I know he has lived longer as a result, but it has been so hard, especially on my mother. Has it made any difference to him?

For now, then, okay: My father is home and here we are. Yet one day soon when my mother has had enough, when my father has become bedridden and mute, when there are no longer any "good" days, my family will have to make other plans: home hospice, 24/7 live-in caregivers, or placement in a nursing home or a dementia unit. Such care may cost more than ten thousand dollars a month, with no insurance buffer. There is no Medicare coverage for long-term custodial nursing-home care, home health aides, dementia units. Yes, hospice will come, in and out, but their services are limited.

What about "long-term-care insurance"? I recently had a patient who had been paying on a long-term-care policy for years. Now he needed help but was doing well in an assisted-living facility. The insurance company refused to pay for any of it, saying that his policy was for "nursing-home care" only. For this man, at this time, his facility was treating him as well or better than any nursing home could. When he took out his policy, there was no such thing as "assisted living," but the company had found some weasel room—and they were taking it.

If your elderly loved one is destitute, he might qualify for some government-sponsored Medicaid assistance. In Texas, the per diem Medicaid reimbursement to long-term-care homes is so low that facilities are often hard-pressed to deliver decent care. Several states are now experimenting with allowing Medicaid to pay for some in-home services rather than only institutional care. Lawsuits have been filed on behalf of elders living in institutional settings demanding that states pay for similar services at home, where people are more comfortable and among family—and the care is actually less expensive and often better. Despite the potential cost-savings in individual cases, the demand for services may burgeon to the point where most states cannot continue this as a viable option. But it makes so much sense, to shift some of these state dollars from institutional to home-care services. Why can't it be done?

Like the doctor whose harangue I have been quoting, there are many who believe that Medicare is responsible for all the ills of our current health-care system. And I am critical as well, especially about Medicare's unjustified excessive reimbursements for "procedures" and "technologies" over "cognitive services." I define these latter services—provided by all physicians, by the way, and not just primary care doctors—as those that entail the thoughtful consideration of a patient's medical story, a complete and full examination, an assessment of all the diagnostic and treatment possibilities in an intelligent, cost-effective way, and a review of all the options with the patient and family. At the risk of repeating myself I must underscore this essential problem of America's medical system: by devaluing cognitive services, Medicare and other third-party payers have—unwittingly but definitely—driven up the cost of health care and deterred many idealistic, compassionate young doctors from choosing a career in family practice, pediatrics, internal medicine, and geriatrics.

This is not the only systemic distortion wrought by Medicare. Just look at what has happened to our hospitals so dependent on government funding. I'm not talking about the slick new doctor-owned specialty hospitals that cherry pick the healthy, less-complex patients away from the big general hospitals, leaving them with those—like the elderly—who require more intensive care and longer stays. The physical plants of our public hospitals deteriorate. Those of us with private health plans see our premiums escalate as cost-shifting goes on behind the scenes to make up for the sub-par payments by Medicare and Medicaid. And now managed-care companies continue to spiral down their payments to providers as well, increasing the speed at which our health-care system circles the drain.

The personnel working in our hospitals are changing as well. There are fewer RNs, and more minimally trained—and therefore less costly—aides or "clinical assistants." These aides may be dedicated, but can we reasonably expect them to deliver the same level of care?

Of course, I am generalizing. The most compassionate people I know work in my hospital. But their ranks are thinning, their pay is poor, their workload is increasing, their benefits are disappearing. Health-care workers who tend the elderly have higher rates of depression—over 10 percent—than any other employed group of Americans. One million RNs will retire by 2010 and our hospitals will be hard-pressed to replace them. Medicare and Medicaid are, in large part, responsible for this: They have cut the heart out of their reimbursements to hospitals. The private insurance companies have followed Medicare's lead. The system is crumbling from within.

And yet I cannot imagine America without Medicare. Think about how many families might be destitute as the result of medical expenses, how many sick old folks would delay getting care until it is too late. Private insurance companies would not rush in to fill the breach if there were no universal health coverage for those over sixty-five. Their practice of excluding people with "pre-existing conditions" (how many folks over sixty-five are perfectly healthy and on no medications?) and their drive for profits guarantee that a majority of our elderly would either be declined for coverage or unable to afford the yearly premiums. The average annual cost of health-insurance premiums for families in Texas today for people who have *not yet* reached the age of sixty-five is $9,100. This figure is almost half the annual income figure considered the federal poverty level.

Medicare, imperfect as it may be, is at least an efficient system with an overhead expense in the range of only 3 percent. Compare this to overhead and profit margins that range from 40 to 60 percent for private heath-insurance carriers, and it is obvious why their premiums are so high. All patients on standard Medicare are treated the same by the system, a real-world example of the ethical principle of social justice. And although it is a government program, it is *not* "socialized medicine." Patients have the right to choose the physician they want from among any of the privately practicing doctors in the community who agree to abide by Medicare's rules. I do not work for the government, even though the vast majority of the patients I see have Medicare coverage. Certainly the current system needs major tweaking—and soon—but it has worked for our seniors for forty years and I, for one, am not in favor of abandoning it. Hopefully, if and when the political debate begins in earnest, the politicians and their policy folks—the ones in charge—will seek out the opinions of those of us on the front lines. This did not happen during previous national debates on this subject.

"Dad, are you happy?" I ask again on that November day.

"Why are you asking me? You should ask your mother."

"I'm asking you, Dad."

My mother says, "Len, you know you're sleeping your life away . . ."

My father is quiet. Maybe he is trying to remember, searching for his forgotten life: his dead mother and brothers and sisters, his return from the war to his bride-in-waiting who wrote to him every day for five years, his two boys snuggled up in his arms for a story at bedtime, his fishing trips out on the Chesapeake Bay, his business looted and gone, his first sighting of a whooping crane at the Aransas National Wildlife Refuge, his artist's soul retrieved and then lost again.

He looks once more at his silver-haired wife. He contemplates my question, looks at my mother again, and then to me. We wait. Finally he answers.

"Sure, I'm happy . . . I have your mother with me. I love your mother, you know." He stares off into the distance.

Even if his memories fail him now, here he is today in his own living room with his wife beside him, no matter how imperfect their life together has been. He truly loves her and she is here, still by his side—frustrated and complaining at times—but still here when he needs her the most.

"I know I sleep a lot," he says. "But I have delicious dreams."

"What?" my mother asks. "What's he talking about?" She is leaning forward in her chair, trying to get a clear look at her husband.

"It's okay, Mom," I say. "It's fine." For a moment my parents search each other's faces.

Outside the window the waxwings tear into the pyracantha berries. My father is suddenly aware of them.

"Look at all the birds," he says. "I planted those bushes, you know."

"I remember, Dad. Would you like to sit outside for a while and get a closer look at the waxwings?"

"Sure," he says. "Don't forget the binoculars, Jerry-boy."

SEVENTEEN

My father is not a religious man. He knows little of Jewish ritual, has no interest in attending organized services. In my lifetime he has been inside a synagogue for his sons' Bar Mitzvahs and for my first wedding. There may have been a few other occasions, celebrations for other family and friends perhaps, but I do not remember them. He is not a "shul guy," as he always said whenever my brother or I offered to take him to a religious service. My father is a loner.

And so I am surprised when he turns to me and asks, "Will you say Kaddish over me?" Kaddish is the traditional Jewish prayer recited in remembrance of a lost loved one. Orthodox Jews recite this prayer at least three times a day in the presence of a *minyen,* a gathering of ten adults, usually in a synagogue. These daily prayers go on for a year, and then once a year at the anniversary of the death. Other Jews recite the Kaddish for much shorter periods of time, a week, or perhaps a month during the traditional mourning or shiva period. Many Jews do not sit shiva at all, preferring to mourn in their own way. I had always believed that my father was this kind of Jew.

Even in his moderate state of dementia he is still able to surprise me. We are sitting together on the old floral-print couch in the living room, its deep blues and greens my father's favorite colors.

"Dad," I say, "is this what you really want me to do? If it is, I'll do it. But you know I will remember you. You know I will think about you . . ."

"I said Kaddish for my father, you know. For a year. Every day."

"Your brothers had to drag you to shul if I remember . . ."

"Yeah," he says. "I wanted to play ball and look at birds . . ."

"Well, you were just a kid then," I say.

"My father died when I was seven." I watch his face; his mind begins to drift, to search. "I can't even remember what he looks like anymore. He used to have a gold pocket watch . . . he'd show it to me sometimes when I sat on his lap. The moon was inside . . ."

"I know," I say.

"Were you there?"

"No, Dad . . . you told me about it. I wasn't born then."

"I get mixed up."

"That's okay, Dad. I understand. And if you want me to say Kaddish for you when the time comes, I will."

"It's a waste of time," he says. His eyes are shining.

"What if I go bird-watching and think of you and all the birds we've seen together?"

"That sounds like a good idea," he says.

He's quiet for a moment, and then, "Take me with you, will you? I don't get out much anymore . . ."

"You'll always be with me, Dad."

My religion tells me that a boy becomes a man when he reaches the age of thirteen, and after a year or more of study—of memorizing the rhythmic chants and melodies from the ancient texts—he ascends the bema on his Bar Mitzvah day to lead the assembled congregation through the Shabbat morning service. He is suddenly alone, this boy-man, as the rabbi, cantor, and all the elders take their seats to listen and to judge.

When it was my turn that Saturday morning in 1961, my chanting reverberated in the stone sanctuary of Beth Tfiloh in Baltimore. I had learned my Torah portions well; my voice had deepened to baritone the year before. I was nervous at first, but after I sang the opening prayer and heard the echo of my own strong notes, I was no longer afraid. I looked up in the balcony where my mother sat with Grandma Bessie and all the other women. I saw her move her mouth and say: "Slow down!"

My father sat close to the front, not far from where I stood above him on the bema. He wore a white skullcap and striped prayer shawl, as did all the men that Saturday morning. I had never seen him in these garments before. He looked suddenly like an old man, surrounded by other old Jewish men. I sang out every note to him, each coarse Hebrew consonant, each wailed vowel. My father did not understand my words; I barely understood the English translation myself. But these ancient melodies summon memories of loss and pain suffered by a people over the millennia. He began to cry. My father knew, as I was only beginning to understand, what life held in store for us both. But on that day neither one of us imagined a time when this father would be unable to recognize his own son. Even now, even as I have witnessed his slow descent into dementia, I am shocked when he does not know who I am. I must quickly wrap myself in the garb of my professional training, retreat into my starched white coat, regain my perspective. Perhaps it would be better if I could just mourn the loss of this father I once knew and get it over with. But I cannot.

After the solemn Bar Mitzvah ceremony there is always a party: wine and food and gifts and flowers and music. In those days, the music was chosen by and for the adults, not the children. My father loved jazz, big band jazz—Benny Goodman and Tommy Dorsey tunes—those songs that raised his spirits through the war years. For the first time I watched, amazed, as he held my mother in his arms and glided as if on air, around and around the ballroom, to "Moon-light Serenade." Smiling, he winked at me over my mother's shoulder every time they drifted past the head table where I sat with my young friends. They could dance, my parents, cool and suave as Fred Astaire and Ginger Rogers. Looking back, I think it may have been the only time I saw them together like this. Joy was not a part of their daily lives. But I saw my father dance that day of my Bar Mitzvah, and it is this vision of him—this happy, even confident man—that I want to remember.

The bookshelves in my father's bedroom are crammed with volumes by Jewish historians, philosophers, novelists: Abba Eban, Golda Meir, Albert Einstein, Isaac Bashevis Singer, Saul Bellow, Joseph Heller, Norman Mailer, Philip Roth. Filled with art by Chagall, Pissarro, Modigliani, Soutine, as well as Cezanne, Monet, Gauguin, Renoir, Picasso, and dozens more. As long as I can remember, there has always been a book—or a pile of them—on his bedside table, or on the covers beside him after he fell asleep.

For the last several months my father has been carrying—even as he pushes his walker he holds on to it—a tattered copy of Bernard Malamud's novel, *God's Grace*. Every page is dog-eared. If I ask him if he is enjoying it, he answers, "I haven't gotten very far . . ." My father clutches *God's Grace* in its torn dust jacket as if it were a talisman.

I am certain that my father's dementia makes it impossible for him to follow a thought from one page to the next; but he keeps reading and re-reading passages from *God's Grace*. Can we ever know what is going through the mind of someone like him, someone whose brain tissue has atrophied, its vital connections knotted and tangled, withered and short-circuited? Still, sometimes something gets through—suffuses his consciousness with meaning, keeps him from giving up completely.

God's Grace is an allegory, a take-off on the biblical creation story. A scientist, the son of a rabbi, finds himself the last man alive after a

thermonuclear exchange between two great powers. Before the ca-
tastrophe he'd been researching at the bottom of the ocean in a one-
man submarine. The scientist surfaces to find a ruined world. Despite
the loss of everyone and everything he once knew and held dear, this
lone surviving man bargains with God, asking that he himself be
spared:

"Please, don't cut my time too short," he begs.

EIGHTEEN

In anatomy lab at Penn I always needed help locating this or that artery or nerve. We all did. Nothing ever looked like the pictures in the text. I remember how my group leaned in around Professor Jean Piatt as he deftly—using only a pair of dissecting scissors—separated fascia from muscle, or dove through omentum and mesentery, pushed fat aside, found what we'd been searching for. "There's your celiac artery," he said.

I spent six months in that lab with Dr. Piatt. He never said a thing about his passion for birding. I came upon his book, *Adventures in Birding: Confessions of a Lister,* quite by accident. It documents his quest to reach the milestone of having seen—"life-listed"—six hundred species of North American birds. The book is chocked with seldom-used words, beautiful and rare as wood warblers: "drisk," "prolegomena," "rodomontade." It's full of wisdom as well, like these lines: ". . . the truly great adventures are within ourselves. Birding is an introduction to this truth. Yes, you have guessed it. Birding is the adventure of one's self." I sent the book to my father on his fifty-third birthday. I was twenty-four then.

"I thought your bird-watching days were over, Jerry-boy, now that you're in medical school," he said to me when I saw him next and he thanked me for the book.

"I'll get back to it one of these days, Dad."

"You can do both," he said. "Let that be a lesson to you."

Once, long after the formaldehyde smell from Gross Anatomy had leached from my skin, I searched out Professor Piatt and asked him why he never mentioned his interest in bird-watching during class. I told him how I, for one, would have loved to learn of his secret passion, to reminisce with him about all the hummingbirds I had seen in Arizona just before I entered med school. He said something like, "Oh well . . . I owed my editor another medical book and luckily for me he agreed to take *Confessions of a Lister* . . ." He seemed almost embarrassed about the book, as if it were not proper material for discussion in the hallowed halls of Penn Med, where scientific research and educating the next generation of practitioners was paramount.

When a medical student at the University of Texas Health Science Center in San Antonio jumped off the tenth-floor observation deck of the hospital, there were only a few lines in the newspaper about it. I remember the murmurings among my colleagues: The student must have been "disturbed"; he must have had "issues." Certainly, went the scuttlebutt, his suicide had nothing to do with his chosen profession. The death of this student—whose name I never knew—had a profound impact on me because it brought back my memories of an old friend.

At the time of this medical student's death I was forty-six years old, with one of the busiest practices in the city. I had been out of medical school for twenty-one years. Despite this lifetime of distance, I thought about the death of my medical school friend, Jake Summer, and was finally able to mourn him as well as this young student I had never met. I was able to mourn the loss of a part of my own self as well.

I can still picture Jake the way he looked the first day I met him, both of us in our short white coats. The pockets of those coats were empty then, but they would soon bulge with stethoscopes and reflex hammers, flashlights, index cards, and assorted notebooks. All we had in the beginning was our enthusiasm and our idealism.

Jake's bushy, almost comical eyebrows overpowered his sensitive brown eyes. You had to study his face to notice those eyes. In our group he was the even-tempered one, the one who never panicked before the exam, the one we looked up to. But there was a sadness about him. I knew his mother suffered from multiple sclerosis and had recently been institutionalized. Though he rarely mentioned it, I'm sure her chronic illness was one reason he went into medicine. But there was no time to talk about that; we had too much to learn if we were to succeed.

Jake, a sweet and gentle man, went into pediatrics. He was a natural.

We were interning in different cities when he took an overdose of sleeping pills. He was gone from my life in an instant and I was still in the middle of that hellish internship year with two more to go. When was I supposed to mourn? When bad things happened during our training years, we were told to take a deep breath and get on to the next case.

We were so exhausted from the long hours, the lack of sleep. During all of these years through medical school, through internship, through residency, we were taught this lesson: You do not matter, your health does not matter, your family does not matter. You may— if it doesn't get in the way of your objectivity—have compassion for your patient. But there is no time, no need for you to have any for yourself.

Jake and I never talked about being brainwashed during our medical school years. We didn't have enough insight, enough perspective, to realize what was happening. Now he is gone and I miss him. Worse, I miss the self I lost along the way, the self it has taken me years to unearth from the morass of those early experiences.

———

Somewhere in that morass, the roots of my eventual divorce from Leslie took hold. Neither of us saw it coming, I believe now, so blindsided we were, so intent in our doctoring lives. But it did come and it was a wrenching time for us both.

I did not expect any support from my own mother and father during this ordeal. I didn't even consider talking to my parents about my troubles until the day I moved out of my home. Reluctantly, I drove over to their house to tell them what was happening. My mother cried and said, "I just want you to be happy."

My father looked at my mother, then at me. I was not soliciting any advice from him, but he had to give it just the same.

"My advice to you," he said, "is to go back home. It's over before you know it anyway."

In his book *The Tennis Partner*, Dr. Abraham Verghese writes about David, a student on his internal medicine rotation, who became his friend. The book chronicles this young man's struggle with drug addiction during his final year of medical school, into his internship, and ending with his suicide. Dr. Verghese reminds us that every year in this country two full medical-school graduating classes—four hundred young doctors—are needed to replace the physicians who kill themselves.

Yes, David had "other issues." Dr. Verghese was a powerfully positive force in this young man's life, but he was unable to save him. Dr. Verghese writes:

> *I cannot help but believe that David's aloneness, his addiction, was worse for being in the medical profession . . . because of the way our profession fosters loneliness . . . The doctor's world is one where our own feelings—particularly those of pain, and hurt—are not easily expressed, even though patients are encouraged to express them . . . we learn empathy, but we rarely expose our own emotions.*
>
> *There is a silent but terrible collusion to cover up pain, to cover up*

depression; there is a fear of blushing, a machismo that destroys us. The Citadel quality to medical training where only the fittest survive, creates the paradox of the humane, empathetic physician . . . who shows little humanity to himself. The profession is full of "dry drunks"—physicians who use titles, power, prestige and money just as David used drugs; physicians who are more comfortable with their work identity than with real intimacy. And so it is when one of our colleagues is whisked away, to treatment, and the particulars emerge, the first response is, "I had no idea."

It is not individual physicians who are at fault as much as it is the system we created.

My friend Jake has been gone a long time. I am still here, still practicing, still basking in the gratitude of many, many people whom I have helped over the years. For this I am thankful. But when I think about the system of medical training in which I was forged, sadness and anger wash over me at unexpected times. Many of us were dehumanized by it, and my fear is that things haven't changed much.

How many physicians today feel a deep unease when we learn that one of our colleagues—even someone we might not know very well—is ill, has had bypass surgery, or has just been diagnosed with cancer or AIDS, or has a "little problem"? How many of us, when we hear that it is one of our own behind a NO VISITORS sign, tiptoe by on our rounds day after day?

In the months after my divorce, before my father became an old, old man, and while my mother was still working in my office, they both somehow understood that I needed them once again. My mother began bringing me a bag lunch every day: a tuna sandwich on rye, a tangerine, some cookies. My father, after years of our mutual disappointment, called me regularly in the evenings, sent me books and articles to read. He took me out to dinner a few times and even picked up the check.

Families can be bastions of strength and comfort despite the fact that almost all of them harbor secrets, deep sadness. I have heard so many stories over the years in the privacy and safety of my examination rooms from the people who have come to know and to trust me. With time they have opened up, shyness giving way to sobbing, trembling. Middle-aged men, tough executives, linebackers in high school, standouts in college, explode in rage, collapse in tears. Sad, sad women encased in heavy makeup wail until there is nothing but the truth left on their faces. We all need a safe place to come home to. Even doctors. Maybe especially doctors.

NINETEEN

The first time Roger Tory Peterson visited Rockport, Texas, was in 1948, the year I was born. His first field guide, published by Houghton Mifflin in 1934—and all those that followed—made him perhaps the preeminent artist-ornithologist of all time. He came to Texas to bird with Connie Hagar, a retired schoolteacher—one of the old old—a passionate, meticulous lister. Despite bad arthritis and cataracts, Connie had documented so many different species in her small coastal community that the bigwigs in the American Ornithologists' Union considered her a nutcase. What she had discovered, of course, was that Rockport lies in the middle of what is now known as the Central Flyway for migrating North American songbirds.

During the years of my doctoring life I have carried my binoculars with me whenever I travel, even to medical meetings. I'd always look for an opportunity to see a new bird. I used to daydream about going birding with Roger Peterson: maybe at Cape May in the spring, spotting plovers, or up in Ramsey Canyon in the summer, looking for bluethroats and broadbills. Perhaps we would listen together for the mournful calls of sandhill cranes at the Bosque del Apache in the fall, or hold our breath as a purple gallinule silently trod over lily pads in the Everglades. Before my binoculars were focused, he'd have found another bird. What a thrill that would be, just trying to keep up, having him by my side.

Throughout his life, Roger visited Rockport often for "birdathons"—folks would donate money to the Audubon Society for each species Roger could find in one long day and night in the field. Once, back in the early nineties, I read in the newspaper that Roger would be in Rockport for one of these events. The photo accompanying the article showed his age: his hair white and thinning, his wrinkled neck. I felt a pang when he admitted in the interview that his hearing was going, especially in the higher registers. "Some birds I just can't hear anymore," he said.

He'd been hard at work on the latest edition of his birding guide. Since 1934 it has sold millions and millions of copies. "The publisher didn't want to take too much of a chance on that first one back then," he said, "so they only printed two thousand copies. I don't even have one myself anymore . . . but I was practically a boy then. How could I know what it would mean to me now?"

In that same interview, Roger said he wished he could fly; he'd often thought how lovely life would be as an albatross, drifting on the air currents above the oceans of the world. So wistful—this octogenarian bird-man really wanting to do that.

The last time my father and I went out into the field together was 1989. He was seventy then; I was forty-one. Our habit, on my first free weekend each spring, was to head for Rockport in the hope that we would catch one of the migration waves. We prayed for a cool front to stall just off the Texas coast. For several nights while the front lasted, the birds overflying the Gulf of Mexico—having left their staging grounds on the Yucatán Peninsula—would "fall out" and pile up in the fields and groves of Live Oak Point, resting and foraging, waiting for calm weather and their second wind before moving north again.

We always drove the back roads. There's an old apple orchard just south of Falls City where we'd look for orioles. In Panna Maria we'd search for scissortails along the hedgerows; just past Goliad we'd scan the coastal prairie for the bobbing heads of sandhill cranes and the occasional swallow-tailed kite diving for insects. Once in a while we'd catch a glimpse of the bald eagle that nested there. Red-tailed and white-tailed hawks, kestrels, and even a rare peregrine falcon stared across the coastal plain from the tops of utility poles as we turned south at Tivoli and headed down the shore road to Rockport.

If we hit it right, the birding was spectacular. "Will you look at that!" my father said, pointing to a salt cedar with six exhausted northern orioles perched in it. A short length of barbed-wire fence might hold an indigo, a lazuli, and a painted bunting. Ten minutes spent scanning the crown of one of the majestic trees out on Live Oak Point might yield ten different species of warblers: black-and-whites, blackburnians, Canadas, Tennessees, yellows, American redstarts, black-throated blues, myrtles, bay-breasteds, prothonotaries, and more. "I can't believe it," my father always said. Those were grand weekends; we'd have a couple of beers, eat fresh filet of flounder, get up early, and go birding again.

I'm not sure why we stopped going. I was busy; he was depressed. Perhaps he didn't feel as if he deserved to enjoy himself. In those years I wanted to spend my precious off-call weekends with my own family, my young daughters. My father and I were still angry and disappointed in each other, though we never talked about it.

In 1994, five years after my father and I had last birded together, I learned that Roger Tory Peterson planned to give the keynote speech in Rockport at the inauguration of the Great Texas Coastal Birding Trail, a project of the Texas Parks and Wildlife Department. Site #1 of this fivehundred-mile highway and trail network begins at the Connie Hagar Cottage Sanctuary in Rockport. I tried my best to talk my father into coming with me. He had just finished his radiation treatments for prostate cancer, wasn't feeling up to par; in retrospect, he was beginning his long, slow decline.

"Come on, Dad," I said. "This is the chance of a lifetime. We might even get to meet Peterson. And we'll do some birding on our own. The hummingbirds and fall warblers will be coming through."

"You go on without me," he said. "I'm too old for that kind of thing now."

I should have been more persistent. I wasn't, and we missed this opportunity—the last one, as it has turned out—to go birding in Rockport together.

Just before Roger Peterson was due to visit Rockport I was hunting through a pile of books at a used-book sale in San Antonio. My good friend, Danny, was on the other side of the table.

"Hey, you like birds," he said. He tossed a slim book across to me.

At first I didn't believe it. The book had a crisp white dust jacket with the words, "*A Field Guide to the Birds . . . A Bird Book on a New Plan* by Roger Tory Peterson." This can't be real, I thought. What sixty-year-old field guide still has a perfect dust jacket? But sure enough, the date on the copyright page was 1934. I planned to give it to Roger after his speech in Rockport.

September 8, 1994, was a hot day on the Texas coast. Roger was eighty-five years old when he walked up the steps of the platform erected on the site of Connie Hagar's former home. Hundreds of people watched: birders, reporters, police and fire personnel, an EMS unit. Roger, hatless, spoke for forty-five minutes in the unforgiving Texas sun. I remember him saying, "There is no such thing as a 'bad' bird.'" He was making the point that in the now competitive world of bird-watching—marathon tournaments where teams compete against one another to list the most species in a limited period of time, or the constant search by the passionate birder for the exotic or "accidental' sighting—we are losing touch with the fact that the birds that surround us every day are marvelous and beautiful creatures, that the house sparrow and house finch, the titmouse and chickadee are every bit as complex and interesting and worthy of notice as any rare bird we might travel far afield to see.

As he was being helped down from the platform, I was admiring the wisdom of his words, thinking about how appropriate they are to the practice of geriatrics. Roger's legs wobbled a little and I watched closely as he was helped to his seat under a canopy, finally out of the sun. People buzzed around him, waving books, wanting his signature. His head suddenly slumped backward over his chair and I saw his body jerk. No one reacted at first, and I began trying to make my way through the crowd toward him.

"Get him on the ground!" I yelled. "Someone get him flat on the ground and lift up his legs!" I hadn't yet seen him take a breath.

Just when I reached him he gasped, inhaled deeply. Then the EMTs sliced their way in, clearing everyone in their path to make way for the gurney. A man in a suit yelling "I'm a doctor, I'm a doctor" and carrying a black bag ran behind them, and before I knew it Roger was whisked off to the nearest hospital. I never did find out what had happened to him that day. He was frail and old but still pushing himself to keep going, not to give in. Roger went home to Old Lyme, Connecticut, and lived two more years. I hope he was able to paint right up until the end.

I wish my father had been with me that day, as upsetting as it might have been for him to see the grand old man of birding taken away in an ambulance.

"What happened to him?" my father would have asked.

"I think it was the heat, Dad. He shouldn't have stood out in the sun that long."

"Will he be okay, do you think?"

"I don't know. He's old and frail now."

"So am I, Jerry-boy," he might have said.

"I know, Dad. We should talk about that, about what you might want when the time comes."

"Let's have a beer. See some more birds in the morning. We'll talk about that stuff some other time."

That time never came.

TWENTY

One morning early in my practice career, I opened the exam room door to greet a new patient. I was surprised to see a nun in her black-and-white habit sitting in the chair, her winged hat perched like a huge seabird on top of her head.

Sister Theo was in her late sixties. She had spent her life serving the community as a teacher and school administrator for the Sisters of the Sacred Heart of Jesus, her religious order. That first time I saw her she had been having abdominal pain for weeks. She'd been to other doctors, but no diagnosis had been made.

As with any new patient—as I was taught from my first day of medical school—I started from scratch with Sister Theo. I asked about the nature of her pain, when it began, the quality of the discomfort, its relationship to meals, position, the presence or absence of triggering or ameliorating factors. I questioned her about her past medical history, including hospitalizations and surgeries, and learned that she had never been sick before. I asked about family medical issues. Despite the fact that she was a nun, I queried her on alcohol consumption and other potentially unhealthy habits. I then began the litany of

questions that doctors call the "Review of Systems"—an extensive inquiry into every bodily system and its function, questions that range
from "Do you ever have headaches?" to "Have you ever experienced
numbness or tingling in your feet?" Many doctors ask their patients
to complete a checklist of these questions before they enter the exam
room. I prefer to ask the questions myself, to observe the patient's body
language as I tick through the list, asking for more detail, explaining
the gist of the questions as I go. The atmosphere of the exam room
is highly charged. All of us will be patients one day and all of us fear
what the doctor might ask, might find, the secrets we may be asked to
reveal, the diagnosis we will, one day, have to accept. In this setting, it
is as important to watch as the patient attempts to answer—that downward glance, that shift in the chair—as it is to hear what is actually said.

Sister Theo was serene and forthright with me even though
some of the things I asked were perhaps embarrassing to her. She
did tell me that she had had some vaginal bleeding although her periods had stopped ten years before. This was an ominous sign. I discovered that she had never had a pelvic examination or a Pap smear,
not even recently, as she had gone from doctor to doctor looking for
help, searching for answers to the cause of her abdominal pain.

Perhaps her previous doctors had decided not to perform a pelvic
exam because of the low incidence of cervical cancer in someone like
Sister Theo. Of course, cervical cancer is not the only reason to examine the reproductive organs of female patients—even in the old and
the old old—on a regular basis. Perhaps they were intimidated or even
embarrassed at the thought of fully examining a nun. Or maybe they
succumbed to wishful thinking, believing that lives spent in contem-
plation of the divine, lives dedicated to educating children and tending to the sick, are lives somehow protected from disease and
degeneration. Doctors are human beings; they can be just as subjective, just as prone to magical thinking, as anyone.

Experimental psychologists study the kinds of errors physicians
are prone to in their clinical decision-making. Given the fact that at

least 15 percent of our initial diagnoses are incorrect, we can certainly use some help. The mistake Sister Theo's former doctors made is known as an "affective error"—a "tendency to make decisions based on what we wish were true."

"Sister," I said after taking her medical history, "I must examine you thoroughly now, including your vagina, uterus, and ovaries. I'll try to be gentle, but I know this will be uncomfortable for you."

"Yes, Doctor. I understand."

I left the room so that my nurse could prepare her. Sister Theo was the first nun I had ever examined, and I was anxious about what I was about to do, but not like the first time in medical school, when my hands shook and my palms sweated as I fumbled with the breasts of a middle-aged woman in the surgery clinic. I was worried about what I might find.

My ability to perform a thorough physical examination has become ritualized through the years. My eyes and ears and fingers work together—intellect and muscle and memory—inspecting, palpating, percussing, auscultating, going back again when something seems amiss or different, remaining attentive to the task, postponing the probing of the tender area to the last. To me, it is a sacred rite, this art of examining the body, passed down through generations of clinicians before me.

Gently I inserted one finger inside her vagina, my other hand pushing down on her abdomen from above. Sister Theo did her best to cooperate, but I could tell from her expression and the tension in her muscles that I was hurting her. I closed my eyes as I always do, focusing my concentration on what my fingertips are telling me. And as I pushed down into her abdomen with the weight of my hand, I felt a hard, irregular mass—something I knew should not be there— bump up against my examining finger.

After I finished and Sister dressed, I sat down with her.

"There is a mass in your pelvis, Sister" I said. "It's most likely a tumor of your uterus or ovary."

"I see," she said.

"Sister . . . it's very possible that this will turn out to be malignant," I said.

"If this be God's will, then so be it," she said. She remained calm—much calmer than I was, than I could ever have been had I gotten this news.

"I'm sorry to have to tell you this today, Sister."

"Thank you for being so kind and so thorough, Doctor," she said.

Sister Theo underwent exploratory abdominal and pelvic surgery that revealed a uterine cancer that had spread throughout her pelvis and abdomen and into her liver.

I first thought to write here that Sister Theo experienced no miracle cure, no divine intervention because, in the end, she died of her disease. Doctors are trained to be results-oriented, to believe that a cure is the measure of our success. This is wrong, of course, but years passed before I realized it. Now, reflecting back a quarter century ago, I remember that Sister did well for many, many months, resumed her teaching responsibilities, and that when her time came, friends and former students and family surrounded her. When I visited her hospital room, she never complained to me, always appeared comfortable, peaceful. As death neared she was free of the angst I have seen so often in my patients, that I witness almost every day in my own father now. Her colleagues kept a vigil by her side, their rosary beads in hand. She died in her sleep and without struggle.

During all the years since I cared for Sister Theo I have had the privilege of serving as the doctor for many nuns in San Antonio. I treat them as I would any one of my female patients. I have prescribed for their diabetes and hypertension, managed their congestive heart failure and strokes, diagnosed their cancers. I have been at their bedsides as they died and have been soothed by the equanimity that I experience when I am with them.

The Sisters who still come to me are all old now; so few young women enter the convents these days. The oldest old are being cared

for by the old old. It was never meant to be this way. In past generations, young, strong women had always been there to care for their aging sisters. They are struggling now, my nuns. Sisters hobbling with
canes accompany those in wheelchairs to my office. Where once their
communities supported their own custodial nursing facilities, some
aging Sisters have had to retreat to fee-for-service secular nursing
homes. Yet they do not complain; they go on doing the best they can.

The School Sisters of Notre Dame, an order based in Minnesota,
have donated their brains to science in unprecedented numbers. The
Nun Study has been ongoing since 1986, when Dr. David Snowdon,
an epidemiologist at the University of Minnesota, first met with Sister Carmen Burg. It was Dr. Snowdon's hope that he could enlist at
least some of the Sisters in a research effort that might eventually
shed light on the aging process. Each enrolled Sister would have to
be open to an examination of her medical and social background, be
willing to undergo extensive neurological and cognitive testing at regular intervals for the rest of her life, submit to blood tests and other tissue sampling, and ultimately, upon her death, allow her brain to be
removed for extensive pathological investigation. Sister Carmen responded to Dr. Snowdon's proposal this way: "We have *always* believed
in the power of knowledge and ideas. A large part of our mission has
always been teaching . . . Our sisters have spent their entire adult lives
trying to help other people in the community . . . I think they would
see your study as a way to continue their lifelong mission of helping
others, of educating others."

This landmark project has been going on for twenty years now and
has contributed significantly to our understanding of Alzheimer's disease. The study has confirmed that this disease is a continuum, that its
roots begin in childhood—the time of most rapid brain development—
when families can provide a rich emotional life and instill an optimistic
outlook that seems to delay the development of this terrible disease. In

adulthood, higher levels of educational achievement correlate with a lower incidence of Alzheimer's dementia.

Dr. Snowdon and his collaborators are confirming gene sequences that code for abnormal amyloid and tau proteins, the substances that accumulate excessively in the brains of Alzheimer's patients. They are correlating brain health or disease with common metals in our environment, like aluminum and mercury; testing hypotheses that vitamins and antioxidants such as vitamin E and C and lycopene and folic acid might be playing a role. The data these scientists produce are powered by the number of enrollees—close to seven hundred— and from the gift of these brain specimens that will be studied and analyzed for years to come.

Of course, when I read about the School Sisters of Notre Dame, I think of all the nuns I have cared for over the years, how many of them live to be among our oldest old; how stalwart they are as they deal with illness, how peaceful during their last days and hours.

Dr. Snowdon has recorded another amazing fact about his group of Sisters: "The risk of death in any given year after age sixty-five is about 25 percent lower for the School Sisters of Notre Dame than it is for the general population of women in the United Sates."

This is a remarkable finding. The reasons for it are purely speculative at this point. But Dr. Snowdon mentions two factors that he believes are important and that I have witnessed in my own association with the Sisters of the Sacred Heart of Jesus.

The first is the deep spirituality common to these women. The second factor that may be contributing to the longevity of these women is the power of community. Snowdon mentions other research confirming a reduction in the risk of death from heart attacks and strokes in adults who maintain strong social connections throughout their lives.

What can we boomers expect as we age? Not many of us belong to religious orders. Will we be better or worse off than our parents' generation? Current Census Bureau figures estimate that by 2030 there will be seventy-two million Americans—one in five—over sixty-five years of age. The good news is that these folks will be the most educated generation in our history—25 percent will have college degrees. We should be healthier as well (if the epidemic of obesity doesn't overtake us): Disability rates have been falling from 26 percent in 1982 to less than 20 percent in 1999. Financially we will also be ahead of the game as poverty rates in the elderly have fallen from 35 percent in 1959 to 10 percent in 2003.

Though it may take us longer to become infirm, we will get old nevertheless. Divorce rates are high, and this, combined with lower birth rates in the boomer generation, does not augur well for the level of family support we will need in our old, old years.

Sometimes, on a good day, I will sit next to my father on his living room sofa, one of his art books opened across our laps. He points to some of his favorite paintings, like Paul Gauguin's mural.

"Oh, I've always loved this one," he will say. But he's forgotten the names of the artists, even the Impressionists whom he admired and tried to emulate.

Years ago when my father and I studied this painting together, I wish that I had not let him close the book on the essential questions the artist asks us to contemplate, but we were both afraid to engage each other on the meaning of life and the subject of death. Most of us are ill-equipped in this regard. The tragedy is that we fail to know each other fully if we refuse to discuss these profound questions. And worse, we fail to fully know ourselves.

My father is a man who—in his own way and in his own time—quests after the meaning of life. Even though he lacks the educational training and tools of formal inquiry, he recognizes the essential questions and is frustrated that he can't formulate his own answers. Somehow—even as a young man—I understood this about him, and there were times as I sat in my college classrooms when I felt his presence, urging me to think, to question, to learn. As his first college-educated son, I rarely found time during my busy doctoring years to engage him on these philosophical issues. In this I failed us both.

When I think about my father's life, there is much that points to his future development of Alzheimer's disease. Here is a man who lost his father at the age of seven, who was raised by a stern, disapproving mother during the Depression, who was removed from high school before graduation, and who was forced to work in a struggling family business. He shunned social connections because of his inferiority complex, lost his business and life savings, and remained isolated and depressed for years, refusing all help and treatment. The miracle may be that he was not demented long before he became an old, old man.

His love of art may have saved him.

Not long ago I was invited to attend a Jubilee Mass of Thanksgiving at the Church of the Holy Spirit in San Antonio. This special service was to honor five Jubilarians—women who had completed fifty years of religious service. I have been the doctor to four of them for many years.

And so I found myself inside a Catholic church—I, a lapsed Jew who has not been to regular services in a decade. I went up to my Sisters, congratulated each in turn. They were dressed in white, corsages pinned to their jackets. These are the youngest left in their convent. Their frail colleagues sat in the front row with their walkers and canes and wheelchairs.

My Sisters stood in front of the priest, their faces relaxed and joyful. I watched as they reaffirmed their vows, took their Communion. I was offered the wafer and wine, but I declined. I'd like to believe in an afterlife. Even some Jewish sects believe in a better world be-

yond, but I cannot. I have spent these last few decades trying in my
small way to prolong life and ease suffering, to help make our existence on this earth a better one.

The ritual I perform is the examination of the human body. It is
a sacred trust—a sacrament—to be allowed to touch and probe another being. A thorough physical examination is the beginning of all
that will follow in the course of the doctor-patient bond, and when
it is done with compassion and respect, it is, by itself alone, a healing
act. No scanner yet invented can substitute for or supplant these hallowed moments. It is in this way that I have tried to fulfill my man-
date as a Jew: *tikkun olam*, to heal the world.

When my Sisters said, out loud and in the presence of all of us in
the church that afternoon, "Lord hear our prayers . . . Inspire others
to join us," I could only murmur in concert with those around me,
"Amen."

Of all the paintings my father produced over the years there are only
two self-portraits. He painted the first one when he moved to Texas
and set up his garage studio. It is from a photograph, a picture I
snapped of him in 1966 during what turned out to be our last fishing trip together on the Chesapeake. Here he is piloting our rented
rowboat. He is wearing his green fishing cap and yellow jacket—and
one of his rare smiles. His hand is on the tiller of our five-horsepower Johnson outboard. A white wake trails off into the blue-green
waters of the bay. His hand, the motor, the details of his face and
clothing—down to the yellow marlin stitched onto the front of his
cap—are all meticulously rendered. This is how he wants us to remember him.

The second self-portrait hangs on the wall directly across from
where he sleeps. It is lit from the lamp on his nightstand. Lying in his
bed, he has the best view of it. In this painting, done twenty years after the first, my father's face fades into a dark blue-green background.

His expression is anguished, tortured. He looks more decrepit in this painting than he does even now that he is one of our oldest old. Ten years ago—when he worked on this, his last canvas—he painted not what he saw but who would become.

We sit together now, father and son on the living room sofa. He is dressed in a gray workout suit and smells faintly of urine. He studies the Gauguin painting in the book open on his lap. His eyesight is still sharp.

"What kind of bird is this?" he asks, pointing to the white bird in the far left corner. I have never noticed it before.

"I don't know, Dad," I say. "It could be an albatross, except for the beak. It looks like a puffin's beak."

"I never heard of a puffin," he says.

"I saw one once in Alaska. I doubt Gauguin ever saw one."

"Don't be so sure," he says. And then he closes the book, grasps Malamud's novel from beside him on the couch, hauls himself onto his feet and into his walker, and begins shuffling back to his bedroom.

I stare at the painting, at this large white bird in the lower left-hand corner. Why is this here? Is it a representation of the Holy Spirit? Gauguin once wrote that the bird represents the "futility of words"—certainly an apt description for the state of affairs between my father and me. Perhaps the bird is an albatross, one of those great seabirds that followed ancient mariners, a metaphor for burdens, a bad omen. Many of us look upon our elderly, on our own impending old age in this way.

I rise from the couch and follow my father down the dark hallway to his room, to his bed with the side rails. He is more unsteady in his walker as each week passes, his body so bent that the device seems to be running away from him as he hangs on for dear life. It is an ungainly dance. My father *is* hanging on for dear life, and he hangs on to Malamud's book, even if it means he will topple as he clutches it instead of the metallic partner designed to keep him up-right. The man who glided through the ballroom at my Bar Mitzvah party, my mother in his arms, will never dance again. He will grasp for *God's Grace* with its words that seem to bring him solace. Clutch it, until it falls apart in his hands.

TWENTY-ONE

My father is falling. His body, stooped and bent, has begun its slow arc back to earth; his muscles, withered and spent, no longer resist the call of gravity. My father is falling through the cracks in his own life. He is falling from grace, plummeting through the remains of his past memories. Perhaps he is falling in love with the ground.

At night he falls between the bed and the three steps to the john. He falls finding his way to the living room. He is tipping over his walker, he is tripping over his feet, he is looking to lean on arms that aren't there. His dreams call to him: He follows the instructions of his dead siblings, his Army drill instructor. He is called by the alarm company to come down to the pawnshop, by the MPs to report to his unit, by his mother to come in for dinner, and on the way he falls. He gets hung up in his nightshirt, tangled in his pants, slips in floppy socks, can't find his shoes because we have hidden them. He falls at the front door calling for his mother, his sisters, his old Army buddies, Nates and Sammy.

And I am failing. I, his son the physician, am failing to keep my father from falling. He forgets to use the call bell on his nightstand. If the bed rails are down, he rolls over in his sleep and falls. If they are up, he somehow manages to crawl over them and falls from an even greater height. He cannot remember that he falls but manages at times to figure out how to finesse the rails: he reaches, pulls the pin, and lowers them before he falls. Or he climbs out at the foot of the bed and then falls.

We must do more, I say. We hire a sitter for the night shift, to be alert to the sounds of my father's rustlings, the light going on, his struggles to lift himself from the horizontal to the not nearly vertical, to keep him from falling. He raves: *Who is this strange person coming into my room in the dead of night? Who is she to tell me there is no need to dress? Who is she to help me to the john? And what has she done with my wife?* My mother is exhausted, trying to sleep a few uninterrupted hours in the next room. *Take me to my wife now!* he demands. *I have to see Frances now!* And my mother is awakened anyway and she gives him another pill, which helps for a while but then only adds to the likelihood he will fall again. So we dismiss the sitter. "It's not your fault," we tell her. "You did your best."

My father is falling, and we, all of us, are failing.

When my father was in the Army Air Corps during World War II, he was unbeatable at Ping-Pong.

He was a lithe young man, a high-school track star, a boy who dove from the railroad bridge and swam across Lake Roland without thinking twice. He was fearless on the football field, throwing himself at the thrashing legs of much bigger players, bringing them down with shoestring tackles. "No one can keep moving if you hit them low enough," he told me when I was just a kid and starting to play football. "Let that be a lesson to you," he said.

In his late teens and twenties, during the years he worked in his family's business and before he was drafted, my father began playing Ping-Pong at the YMCA in downtown Baltimore. A leftie, he held his racket with three fingers around the handle, his thumb and index fingers snaked up along the paddle's edges. He had no one to coach him but over time developed a style that confounded his opponents.

In my mind's eye I see him playing, a gangly young man in Army fatigues, pale gray eyes behind wire-rimmed glasses—"Winnie," his buddies called him—taking on all comers. His opponents flew in on prop planes from other battalions, GIs, like my father, who were passing time between their shifts loading gasoline cans onto ships bound for Patton's Army as it barreled across Europe, or waiting to be sent over themselves. The soldiers crowded around the table, urging my father on with their bravado, the smoke from their ration of Lucky Strikes and Camels filling the barracks. They put down their pay and their packs of cigarettes, betting on their pal Winnie to keep slamming those little white balls down the throats of his opponents. He was a star then, center stage, bounding back and forth, paddle flashing in front of him, fielding each volley, reversing the spin, returning the ball low over the net, smashing it home.

Maybe these were the best years of his life, though he would never say so: away from home for the first and last time, out in the wider world, away from the family he loved but from whom he received so little respect or encouragement. Back then he was a winner.

I remember how proud I was of him, hearing these tales in the days before I could even hold a Ping-Pong paddle in my own hand. "So you were the Army champion of all time?" I asked.

"No, no," he said. "Eventually they found someone who beat me. Strangest thing I ever saw . . . a real tall guy, held his paddle upside down, hit the ball from underneath the table, it seemed . . . I never could figure out where the thing was coming from, couldn't gauge the spin. He beat me bad. And let that be a lesson to you," he added, "no matter how good you think you are, there's always someone better."

"Can we get a Ping-Pong table?" I asked. In those days we lived in a tiny second-story apartment.

"One day we will," he said.

My father made good on this promise. In 1953 my parents

bought their first house. My father, back fewer than five years from the war, had reopened the family pawnshop and gone hat-in-hand to his uncle, a wealthy banker, seeking a loan for the down payment. This uncle, who died years later, leaving millions to charity, laughed at him. "You'll never get a loan," he said. With the help of the Federal Housing Administration and Grandma Bessie, my father bought the house on Forest Park Avenue at a cost, I remember, of fifteen thousand dollars. It must have seemed like a fortune to him.

Just beyond the breakfast nook a door opened onto a narrow staircase that led down to a dank concrete basement. Pretty soon my father, using only hand tools and working late into the nights and Sundays, began to transform this space. He built a wall of knotty pine storage closets along one side of the basement, and opposite them a set of bookcases. He installed fluorescent lights in a paneled ceiling, laid green tile on the floor. There was a ground-level window at the far end of the basement and there he built a mini aviary where canaries sang and parakeets chattered. I loved watching him work; he showed me how to use a level, saw a board, drive a nail. One day I came home from school to find a Ping-Pong table in the center of the room.

So began our rivalry. Each night, as soon as dinner was finished, I'd start nagging him.

"Come on, Dad, let's go down and play!" He was patient (there is nothing more boring for a good player than to volley with a novice), hitting balls back and forth with me, teaching me about spin and counter-spin, the art of feinting and dropping the ball just over the net, how to blow a serve past your opponent, how to bring the paddle over the top of the ball, slamming it back across the table should he manage a return. "The old one-two punch," he called his blazing serve followed by his powerful slam.

Through junior high and high school I kept getting better and better. I beat all my friends and the other neighborhood kids. I could never beat my father. He never let me win—until I went off to college and came home during sophomore year. I'd been minoring in Ping-Pong that semester because there was a table just one floor down from my dorm room. I finally beat my father a few times but never consistently. "I see my money is being well spent up there in that college," he said.

He was forty-eight years old then and I was nineteen. Except for his Sunday gardening he was a sedentary shopkeeper, yet he could move back and forth behind that table as well as I. By the time I was forty-eight I hadn't held a paddle in my hand in over twenty-five years.

There is an old barn with a concrete floor on our small ranch outside of San Antonio. A few years ago I set up a Ping-Pong table there. My father was still walking without assistance then, though a steady hand was always nearby. One Sunday my brother, Michael, drove my parents out to the country and he sat them down to watch us play. My father was smiling and following our game intently. "Good shot," he said. "Nice volley." He was then eighty-one years old and hadn't played Ping-Pong since I was in college.

"Dad, you want to play?" Michael said. He was kidding, of course, but my father stood up. "Sure," he said. I knew this was crazy, but when I saw the look on my father's face I couldn't say no.

I looked at Mike and he nodded as if to say, "Don't worry." He handed my father the paddle but moved only a half-step behind him. My father steadied himself and got ready to serve me the ball. He had a fierce glint in his eye, an almost wicked smile. He stared down the table's white sideline as if he was going to serve it there. Suddenly the ball came low over the net in the opposite direction and I lunged to return it. I'd forgotten this old trick of his and barely managed to lob the ball back. He swung at it hard to slam it back but missed, spun around, and would have fallen if my brother hadn't anticipated the whole scenario and caught him in his arms.

"I can't play anymore," my father said.

"That was a hell of a serve, Dad."

"If I played as much as you, I'd beat you every time," he said.

———

Why do we fall when we get old? What happens that draws us back to the ground? Why this reversal of evolution, this surrendering to a lifetime of gravity's invisible tug? First the canes render us tripeds, and then we become multi-legged as the walkers roll out. The wheelchairs follow and we slither, mollusk-like, toward the bed, toward the box, toward the grave. But why do we fall?

Our eyes fail and the floor beneath our feet retreats into shadow, appears as if at the bottom of a dark ocean. Perhaps we can no longer feel, our feet numb to pressure or pain, as if they are anchors encased in iron. We fall because the tiny canals in the inner ear that, like tiny gyroscopes, monitor our position from the vertical, atrophy and calcify, sending false signals to the part of the brain that deciphers them. We reel, we list, we spin like a ship at sea in a storm, about to capsize. Perhaps the brain itself, where all the instrumentation is monitored— speed and wind, stars and tides—shorts out and we are rudderless.

Our muscles atrophy and our joints freeze and our bones become brittle and weak. We fall and break our hips, or our weak hip bones crumble from the weight of a life, and then we fall.

We may lose consciousness to a sudden dearth of blood and oxygen when our pumps fail or short-circuit or go too slow. Our circulatory pipes may be rusted, encrusted with debris that impedes the flow, or loose fragments fly downstream, landing in the nether parts of our control box, a monkey-wrench cast into the engine of our neurological works.

We fall because our bodies no longer make the neurochemicals that lubricate and facilitate the cellular transmissions from brain to nerve to muscle. We are stiff as ungreased cogs, unable to move except in trembling half-steps, halting lurchings that take us nowhere but toward the horizontal.

Most often we fall from a combination of all of these—"a multifactorial gait abnormality," the neurologists say. My father, his cataracts long removed, sees perfectly—"old eagle-eyes," my mother calls him. She can't make out my face unless I put it right up to hers. If she drops her hearing aid or her glasses or the TV remote, she must get down on hands and knees and feel around, unless my father is in the room.

"I'll get it," he says, forgetting that he cannot get up by himself, walk unassisted, or bend over without falling flat on his face.

"Don't move!" my mother yells. "Just tell me where it is." He does. They are bound in a mutually beneficial and sustaining relationship that many couples, long together, participate in without even knowing it, a relationship that often ends in the quick demise of the remaining partner after the first has departed.

My father will continue to fall until the day he dies unless he becomes bedridden and immobile as a result of a debilitating stroke. As long as he continues his struggle to stay upright—to stand, to walk— he will be at risk of falling. No matter the walker, the supporting arms, the hospital bed, the grab bars in the bathroom, even the wheelchair—as long as my father has the will and desire to seek out my mother's face in the next room, to come into the kitchen for the comfort of a meal, to sit in front of the TV and watch a forward pass or a home run, he will be at risk and he will fall.

Our elderly will fall if we allow them the least opportunity to remain independent—yet isn't this a goal worth striving to achieve? When I first entered private practice and began caring for patients in nursing homes, I was appalled at the steps these facilities took to prevent their residents from falling. Old men and women were tied to their beds, rails up, restrained at the wrists or posey-belted around the chest. In their nightly struggles they slipped between the mattress and the railings and sometimes suffocated, or worked their belts around their necks and hung themselves in their own beds. When they were allowed into the hall at meal time, they were placed into a sturdy seat with a sliding tray—like a baby's high chair—that locked into place. There they sat for hours, their heads slumping over into their food. All this was done, and is still done in some places, so that our grandparents, our parents, could avoid a fall.

"Fall cases"—as they are called by the medical malpractice attorneys—are common today, their numbers increasing. These cases are often worth millions of dollars because punitive damages may be awarded if "neglect and abuse" can be proven. I have been called as an expert witness on occasion to testify in these cases. "I've got a fall case I'd like you to look at, Doctor," the voice on the other end of the line will say.

The stories, as they are related to me, are remarkably the same. Old granddad was doing just fine until he was admitted to the nursing home where "they let him fall, he broke his hip, and he died." Then the records come, box after box, shipped "Priority," the patient's medical history often going back for years.

In 2001 I reviewed the story of Mr. Horace Peel, a patient who reminds me very much of my father. He was an elderly man with chronic heart disease and dementia, admitted to a nursing home. He was often agitated and belligerent and had fallen many times at home. X-rays showed healed fractures of both wrists, as well as other broken bones from past falls. In the nursing home he was cared for by an internist and a geriatric psychiatrist who attempted to manage his dementia with medications rather than physical restraints—the conventional, enlightened standard in long-term-care practice today. Despite the best efforts of the nursing-home staff, Mr. Peel fell on several occasions, sustaining only minor injuries. The family insisted on physical restraints, including a posey or vest restraint, although this was contrary to the recommendation of the facility's Restraint Committee. Finally, despite all of this, Mr. Peel fell in the shower room with an aide in attendance, fracturing his hip. Often, it is the osteoporotic, brittle hip bone that gives way and causes the fall, but the two events—the break, the fall—happen so close in time that it is difficult to prove which came first.

The hip was repaired and Mr. Peel lived two more years, eventually dying of his heart disease but not before being transferred to another nursing home where he fell yet again, fracturing his arm despite wearing a restraint device that he managed to remove. The case against the first nursing home and the doctors was settled for a large sum.

There are so many bones to break—wrists and arms and ribs and vertebrae, shoulders and elbows and hips and knees. I receive glossy brochures from a local hospital touting their expertise in bone and joint repair. Here they showcase the assembled team: four young, buff orthopedists (one of the most sought-after specialties in medicine today) wait in surgical greens, well trained, eager. There is so much to be done, so much technology: fiber optics and lasers, titanium and steel alloys, robotically manipulated interventions, tissue-friendly cement and adhesives.

Our medical-industrial complex is enraptured with our falling elderly. What a huge economic force they have become: One in three people over the age of sixty-five falls each year; 10 to 15 percent suffer serious injury with a price tag of over $20 billion paid primarily by the Medicare system.

Often the old folks are out of the hospital before the geriatrician even hears about the fall. They're sent off to the rehab facility where they endure hours each day of physical therapy, occupational therapy, group therapy. They are given pain meds and muscle relaxants and sleep meds, antianxiety meds and antidepressants. They become somnolent or confused, incontinent or constipated from all the drugs, develop unremitting diarrhea from the antibiotics, or spike a temperature from the aspiration pneumonia they got from being too sleepy to swallow. Perhaps they become septic from a skin infection at the operative site, or in the urinary tract as a result of the Foley catheter, or in the replaced joint itself where the foreign body—the titanium invader—now lurks. And now the Medicare benefits for skilled nursing care have run out because the patient—in the words of the bureaucracy—is "no longer making progress."

The call comes from the surgeon to the geriatrician: "To which nursing home would you like us to transfer your patient?"

———

When my first wife and I moved to San Antonio in 1973 for our residencies, we found a small apartment. We rented two rooms of furniture and began looking for odds and ends to complete our living space. This is how we met Evelyn Todd.

Evelyn had an antique shop in Boerne, Texas, a little town about thirty miles north of San Antonio. She was an outgoing woman with a full head of white hair. Her blue eyes had a glint of mischief. She entertained us with her extraordinary tales of travel all over the continent, in search of the "junk"—as she called it—she sold in her shop. The first time we were in the store my wife spied an old brass desk lamp, green with corrosion, the wiring brittle and frayed.

She picked it up and brought it to the counter. "Will this lamp work?" she asked Evelyn.

"I tell you what," Ms. Todd said. "If you clean the brass, I'll rewire it for you."

"How much?" I asked.

"Can't say 'til I see how much time I've got to put in it," she said.

We took the lamp home and worked over its surfaces with Brasso, rubbing off the corrosion, layer by layer. Our fingers were stiff and sore from the effort. It was over a month before we took the lamp, now shiny as new, back to Evelyn's shop. She looked at it and then at us, shook her head. "Well I'll be damned. I'll see what I can do," she said.

More weeks passed before we got back to Boerne and Evelyn's store. The lamp was sitting on the counter, rewired, topped with an antique glass shade and brass finial.

"Um, I'm not sure we can afford it right now . . ." I said.

"It's yours," she said. "I figure anyone willing to work that hard cleaning a piece of old junk ought to just have it."

When I opened my practice a few years later, Evelyn became my patient. I got to know her family. For almost thirty years we celebrated occasions together: my daughters' Bat Mitzvahs, a wedding, her seventieth birthday.

"I never thought I'd make that one," she said. She brought us baskets of apples from her yearly jaunts to the mountains of New Mexico. She kept her shop full of interesting things. We'd come by at Christmas and sing carols together.

From years of hard work—lifting heavy antiques in and out of her pickup truck and on and off the shelves of her shop—Evelyn wore herself out, joint by joint. Both hips were replaced and then the right one had to be replaced again. She refused to let her increasing frailty slow her down. At eighty-five she had a fourth operation, a second left hip repair. It didn't go well; she developed an infection in the joint. After this I had to maintain her on daily antibiotics to keep the infection under control; she insisted that she would have no more surgeries. The chronic drugs caused recurrent bouts of diarrhea.

The pain began to wear her down. She sold the shop. She could no longer drive, then needed a wheelchair. She was falling at home, her muscles weakened by inactivity and chronic pain.

"You need a stronger pain medicine," I told her again and again.

"I don't want to be hooked on drugs," she said.

"Evelyn, look at you!" I finally cried out in frustration. "I can't stand to see you suffering like this. Let me give you something. There's no shame in this. That's what the medication is for."

Eventually she relented, but the drugs affected her mental acuity and she slept more and more. We both knew that her life, as she wanted to live it, was over.

She fell one last time, just past her eighty-ninth birthday. Her infected left thigh bone splintered like a stick of termite-infested wood. She was brought into the emergency room by ambulance and I came to see her.

"We can try to fix this again, Evelyn," I said.

"No," she said. "I'm ready."

There was to be no more slicing through skin and muscle. No more sawing through bone. No more chiseling and tapping, scraping and cementing. No more stainless-steel planes and hammers, drills and screws. No more physical therapy consults, exercise routines, walkers and canes. There was only Evelyn, in her white-sheeted hospice bed, an intravenous line for morphine, and a family: sad, stalwart, and loving. It didn't take long.

I will always miss her.

And my own father? He still struggles to stay upright. He pushes his walker back and forth from bedroom to living room to kitchen. He teeters; sometimes he topples. So far he has not broken anything, but I fear it is just a matter of time.

During the day, my mother and Yolanda keep a constant eye on him. My brother and I always have a hand ready to steady or catch him. But he wanders in the night—to the john, to the kitchen, to check on my mother. Who knows why he journeys? He is on his own at these hours; by morning he forgets ever having embarked on these nighttime travels. He will not be deterred from his nocturnal ramblings, as if he is certain that—in these quiet hours after the moon has risen—he will finally find what he has lost.

Perhaps he searches for the door that will take him down into the club basement where his young son waits for him behind the green expanse of the table, on the other side of the net, a paddle in his hands.

TWENTY-TWO

February 24, 2006, is my parents' sixtieth wedding anniversary. My family plans a brunch for them in their home. We are keenly aware that this may be the last anniversary my parents will celebrate together. It won't be an elaborate party, just a bittersweet one.

I was sixteen when my grandma Bessie and her husband, Sam, celebrated their fiftieth anniversary. It was a real occasion, loads of people, mounds of food. My grandmother wore a white satin gown that only accentuated her yellow skin. Within a few months she would be gone, her pancreatic cancer relentless, but she stood tall as she welcomed her guests.

"I want you should all have a wonderful time," she said. "I want you should eat all this delicious food. You shouldn't think about anything else but having a good time."

I knew my grandmother was dying. I could eat nothing and hid in an upstairs bedroom until I—embarrassed in the face of her bravery—was able to compose myself again.

Bessie died at age seventy. My mother is still ticking along at eighty-one. She is a breast cancer survivor. After the surgery, after the bandage came off, she looked down at herself and said, "It's not so bad." She has severe macular degeneration, adult-onset diabetes, and arthritis. She is deaf. She will say, however, that her greatest disability is my father.

For a week or two before their anniversary celebration, I remind my father about it whenever I visit. "Do you know what's coming up real soon?" I ask. "A special occasion."

"No," he says.

"Does the date February twenty-four mean anything to you?"

"Sounds familiar . . . What is it?

"Your wedding anniversary, Dad. Sixty years you'll be married to Mom."

"I don't believe it," he says. "I love your mother, you know."

"I know you do."

I do know this. I've known this since I was a child, known it despite the angry words I heard on so many occasions. Afterward, my mother would be silent for days; my father, never blameless, would always relent, seek her forgiveness. The arguments were never really about the triggering incident—the unneeded purchase, the forgotten birthday, the messy bathroom—but always about something else entirely, some unnamed grievance, a deep, basic misunderstanding between them. I never heard my mother say, "You know, Len, when you say those things to me, you hurt my feelings terribly!" I never heard my father say, "Fran, I'm sorry. Let's sit down and talk about how this all got started so we can clear the air."

This pattern of noncommunication is common in many marriages, especially in my parents' generation before self-help books and talk therapy became popular. My mother wanted a father-protector; my father wanted a woman to love him with overt affection and quiet passion. Each knew what the other wanted, but they were unable to give it. I, their son—the one always in the middle—tried to make it right.

I realize from my long experience of dealing with other families that mine could have been much, much worse. I love my parents even though I still harbor some disappointment in them about how they lived their lives, how I eventually became—with their assent and approval—a substitute father to them both. I believe that given their own upbringing and limited opportunities for self-enlightenment they did the best they could.

As I have watched my parents grow old together, I see what love means when life is waning, what love finally comes down to as we grow old with our life partners, descend together into disability and, for some, dementia. And as strange as it may seem, I am learning about this from my elderly parents, one blind, one demented.

A few days before they are to celebrate their sixtieth wedding anniversary, my mother calls me in a panic. My father is bellicose and paranoid. He accuses her of all sorts of betrayals; he curses at Yolanda in Yiddish, strings of foreign profanities he has not uttered in seventy-five years. He will not be bathed or shaved. He will not eat, refuses his medications. He is raving.

"Dad," I say, "what is it? What's wrong?"

"I want to go home. Please, take me home!"

"But, Dad, you *are* home."

"I don't know where I am. Please, Jerry-boy, take me home. You know the way . . ."

"I don't know where else to take you, Dad. You've lived here for twenty-nine years."

"You go to hell! You're in with them!"

"Don't talk that way to your son, Leonard!" my mother says. "You're out of your mind!" There are tears in her eyes.

"You go to hell, too, you, you lying bitch, goddamn bitch!"

For an instant I am transported back in time. My first instinct is to protect my mother. I have been bred by her to rise to her defense, confront my father, back him down, even if he hadn't been the one to start the argument. It is a game I stopped participating in decades ago. "You two deserve each other," I learned to say. And then I would leave. They stewed. My mother was silent, refused to cook for a day or two. The next time I saw them, everything would be as it had always been—at least on the surface.

There is no walking away now. My father is demented. His agitation and paranoia arise from distorted memories, nightmares he can no longer separate from reality. He is an abandoned child. He searches for his boyhood home on Boarman Avenue, or perhaps our first house in Forest Park. He hears voices but can't decode what is being said and his mind assumes the worst: My mother is insulting him, planning to run off; his sons are belittling him, his mother scolding him, his older brothers and sisters teasing him. He is lost, with no father to turn to. I see that he has wet himself; a dark ring marks his place on the couch.

My anger melts away. I have been through this before—not only with my father but with many of my patients over the years. I have been cursed, spit on, bitten, pinched, and punched by demented old folks over the decades. A poor woman threw a shoe at me when I stepped inside the door of her hospital room. The day before, she thought I was the devil.

I assume my doctor role with my father; I retreat once again into the armor of my starched white coat. As a doctor I know what to do; as a son I am uncertain. "Talk therapy" will not work here; the time for psychoanalysis, for delving deep into his life has long since passed. It is time to acknowledge his fears at the moment, to let him know I will do whatever I can to ease his agitation.

"Dad," I say, "you're all upset. Let me get you something that will help settle you down." I look into his eyes, now wild with suspicion, with fear. I pat him on the thigh. I take his hand in mine. He does not pull it away. I feel his pulse. It is strong and even. "I love you, Dad. Wait here just a minute."

I walk the few steps to the kitchen and check the daily pill slots

to make sure he's been getting his regular medications. Sometimes my
mother, unable to see, inadvertently leaves pills in the plastic containers
I fill every couple of weeks. But now everything seems in order.

My father takes eight medications a day; my mother fourteen.
They are both on vitamins and minerals, blood pressure medications,
diuretics, and cholesterol-lowering drugs. My father also takes two
pills for his heart. My mother takes drugs for her diabetes, a thyroid
disorder, osteoporosis, and an antidepressant. This is not unusual for
folks their age.

I spend my doctoring days prescribing medications for my patients, re-shuffling the ones they're on—a tiny dose change here, a re-
timing of administration there. By now I have written or refilled
hundreds of thousands of prescriptions, but my constant goal is to cut
back on medications, stop them altogether if I can: Less is usually
more. Every geriatrician knows this. All of us have witnessed the negative effect of "polypharmacy" in our patients. By simply taking the
time to spread all the drug bottles out on the desk, noting each one,
thinking a few moments about the patient and her symptoms, and
saying: "Quit taking this drug!" we can often bring about a rapid improvement in a patient's condition.

I'll never forget Lilly, a middle-aged woman who had taken a two-
hour bus ride to see me and carried a brown paper shopping bag
crammed with pill bottles—at least forty different drugs prescribed by
a dozen physicians.

"This one's for the high blood," she said, "and this one's for the
sweet blood and this one's for the low blood. These three are for my
bad knees and this one's 'cause I'm sad a lot and this one's 'cause
I don't sleep too good and this one's 'cause I'm tired all the time . . .
I can hardly keep 'em straight, but I got a big list at home tacked to
the wall over the phone in my kitchen. Last month the company cut
off the service when I couldn't pay the bill. All these medicines and
still I feel so bad. That's why I come to you now. That and all these
other troubles." She handed me a list of symptoms, pencil-scrawled
on a ragged piece of paper.

I give every new patient an hour of time. I spent two hours with Lilly but felt I had just scratched the surface. She went on and on, one story looping into another, family troubles, bad marriages, kids in jail, all interspersed with medical encounters, ER visits, hospital stays, surgeries, strange diagnoses mostly self-made, aches and pains, hostility, and tears.

I knew what was happening to Lilly, what happens to many people like her in the real time of a medical encounter. The physician begins to drown in a sea of conflicting information, begins to doubt the veracity of the patient's story, feels powerless to alter the circumstances of this person's life. A wave of helplessness washes over doctor and patient both. The physician reaches for his prescription pad, the power he has that she does not, the power to prescribe. "Here, try this," he says. "I think it will help. If it does, I've authorized refills for you." The encounter is over; the doctor steps into the hall and closes the door. He takes a deep breath, picks up the next chart, and prepares to apologize for running so behind in his schedule. He moves on, tries to forget about that last patient, hopes the drug he prescribes will help but doubts it, hopes she will find another doctor next time.

The patient, now alone in the exam room, removes the paper gown, dresses herself slowly. She had so much more to tell this doctor; she was so hopeful that he might help. He seemed like a nice man; her neighbor had seen him once and said he had helped her. Doctors are very busy, yet he did seem interested in her, spent more time than usual. She picks up her bag, heavy with the half-forgotten portable contents of her life, and glances at the desk where just moments ago the doctor sat. On it lies the small square of paper with her name and today's date. She cannot read the other words; it is in an illegible hand, a foreign tongue. It is a potion, a promise, maybe even a cure. She did like this doctor. He listened longer than most. She scoops the paper off the desktop, shoves it into her purse, and vows to make a new start.

When Lilly left my office after that first visit, I had whittled her medication list down to five. After her second visit, after I had obtained some lab work and some old records—and after spending another forty-five minutes—she left my office on only three. I could not change the circumstances of Lilly's life, I couldn't make up for her poverty and lack of education, for the poor choices she had made, or her bad luck. Lilly was always going to be a challenge for me, for any doctor, but she improved so much off all those drugs, was so much more energetic, so much more alive, that I had to pat myself on the back. Even so, I admit, I tried to dodge a long-term commitment to her.

"Lilly," I said after another forty-five-minute follow-up visit that should have taken fifteen, my nurse knocking on the door, giving me the signal that my other patients were getting impatient, "you're so much better now, and I know how hard it is for you to get out here on the bus. Maybe we can find you a physician closer to your home?"

"Oh, no, Doctor . . ." she said. "I wouldn't change from you for the world. Besides, I save so much on my medicine bill I can afford to take the taxi."

Lilly died under my care, at an old age, from heart disease. We went through a lot together before the end came.

Prescribing for the elderly is complicated. They don't metabolize drugs at the same rate as younger, healthier patients. The main work-horses of drug excretion—the liver and kidneys—decline in function with age, as do all our organ systems. The elderly, like my parents, are often on multiple drugs (including over-the-counter preparations the doctor might not even know about) and the incidence of unto-ward drug-drug interactions begins to mount. We know so little about these interactions. Indeed, the pharmaceutical companies are infamous in geriatric circles for not including our elderly patients in drug trials where these problems often (but not always) come to light.

These days, between the Food and Drug Administration (FDA) and Big Pharma, I hang suspended in a netherworld of prescribing angst. The FDA has pulled more than twenty drugs off the market in the last two decades, drugs they first assured me were safe to use but then ended up damaging livers or kidneys or hearts. I have always tried to protect my patients, wait if I possibly can, for after-market studies to bring more data to light. It is one thing, I tell my patients, to judge a drug's benefits and risks after it has been given to a few thousand patients in clinical trials; quite another after it has been prescribed to hundreds of thousands upon its general release.

In the parlance of the technology and pharmaceutical industries, doctors like me who are cautious, who do not immediately jump on the company bandwagon every time it trumpets its "latest and greatest" product, are known as "slow-adopters." Now they have figured out a way to circumvent my judgment should I fail to join the chorus of cheerleaders for their latest breakthrough. On television, in magazines, they promise an end to arthritis pain, a good night's sleep, a cure for incontinence, a firm erection. My phone rings off the hook; some patients feel I am blocking their path to the Fountain of Youth when I decline to prescribe a drug they have been convinced by an effective ad campaign that they must have. Some even change doctors, to one more pliable in this age of consumer-directed medical care.

I have no sympathy for Big Pharma, as you might understand, even when a jury in Texas awarded mega-millions of dollars in damages to the family of a seventy-one-year-old man—a long-time patient with heart disease—who succumbed to a heart attack. He took Vioxx for less than a month before he died. Do I believe that Vioxx was the culprit? I doubt it. Indeed, the maker of Vioxx is being sued over and over by plaintiffs across the country—they are winning some cases, losing others. They have vowed to fight each case. Our justice system often fails to ferret out the real truth in situations like this. But I resent the intrusion of Big Pharma into the doctor-patient relationship, resent the constant introduction of new—often rushed—products into a marketplace crowded with me-too drugs. Big Pharma is right where they have always wanted to be—smack-dab in the middle of my decision-making process as they try to directly influence consumers who also happen to be my patients. Now that they are where they are, they can expect only more litigation as the drugs they hawk on national TV do not live up to the claims made about them.

And yet here I am in the kitchen of my parents' home, rummaging through a basketful of medicines I take down from a high shelf. Here is where I store the unused pills—all the psychoactive drugs previously prescribed by my father's physician for his recurrent bouts of anxiety or agitation, for his depression and his insomnia, for his memory loss and lethargy, for his confusion and paranoia, for his belligerence and sadness.

I take down a dozen orange plastic pill bottles with white almost-impossible-to-remove lids. My father's name is on every label: Some are six months old, some several years. We have been dealing with this for a long time.

Haloperidol and risperidone. Olanzapine and quetiapine. Paroxetine and citalopram. Alprazolam and trazodone. Donepezil and rivastigmine and memantine. Organic molecules, various combinations of carbon and hydrogen and nitrogen, oxygen and sulfur—the atoms of which we are all made—bioengineered to slip across the blood-brain barrier, to stimulate one receptor or block another, precipitate a rush of ions through neural membranes, flood synaptic gaps with potent neurotransmitters, flip a switch here, throw a breaker there, block a surge somewhere else . . . all to make us whole again, to bring us back to our senses, to jump-start us once more.

It is an act of faith for me to prescribe any medication and an even greater act of faith for my patient to fill the prescription—much more expensive than it ought to be—and then swallow it, take it inside, day after day, often year after year. I know that I am the professional, the "scientist." It is my role to evaluate these drugs, vet them, understand their pharmacology, their interactions, their effects on physiology, their complications. I am the one licensed by the state to make these choices, monitor these therapies. I am the captain of the ship, the one responsible if things go wrong.

But now any physician who prescribes these "atypical antipsychotic drugs" for his elderly patients does so at his peril. The Food and Drug Administration—after first granting approval—has recently withdrawn its blessing for these medications in the treatment of behavioral disorders in our elderly folks with dementias. For years geriatricians and psychiatrists used these drugs with some success. Medications like risperidone rendered perhaps a 20-30 percent benefit potential—often when nothing else would—when weighed against a 2 percent chance of serious peril.

Who should I believe when conflicts of interest so bedevil the institutions I must depend upon? Medical scientists whose grant monies spur them to turn a hypothesis about a class of organic chemicals into advancement and tenure and, nowadays, a piece of the action? My doctor colleagues who reconfigure their offices into lucrative clinical research mills, abandoning patient care except as a means to recruit the naïve, the unsuspecting, the uninsured who are desperate for free medications or the money they receive for "guinea-pigging" in drug trials? Big Pharma, wily and flush with incentives, promoting the next breakthrough as if every one was as miraculous as penicillin? The FDA, Big Pharma's enabler, assuring me that all is well, stamping its seal of approval on the drug? That is, until they remove it again, after I finally relent, buy into the hype. Frantically we try to track down patients, alter medical regimens, pray we haven't hurt anyone.

And whom are *you* to trust? If you have a copy of the *Physician's Desk Reference,* if you go online, if you read the information that comes—mandated by law—from the pharmacist, would you ever put a drug like risperidone in your mouth or in the mouth of your loved one? Here are but a few of the side effects you might experience from the first dose or the thousandth: low blood pressure and thus a tendency to fall or pass out; impairment of judgment and/or motor skills; tardive dyskinesia (a potentially irreversible involuntary movement disorder); neuroleptic malignant syndrome (a sometimes fatal reaction: high fever, muscle rigidity, sweating, altered mental states, and cardiac arrhythmias). Of course, some of these are very rare and therefore quite unlikely to occur, but at the same time they are entirely unpredictable.

Nevertheless I am in my parents' kitchen searching for the bottle of risperidone tablets so that I can give one to my father, so that I can review with my mother how to use it during the times he is belligerent and agitated. Although I am reluctant to use this drug—any drug—in treating my father, I often resort to them for two reasons only.

The first and foremost rationale, I tell myself, is that I have used it before in my father with success. It has worked. It has settled him down, albeit with an added degree of cognitive impairment he can ill afford.

The second reason is that I hope by using this drug—judiciously and in a closely monitored fashion—I can maintain the status quo and keep my father at home for a bit longer; because, in my judgment, the risk to my father in a long-term-care facility is greater than the risk of asking him to swallow another risperidone tablet.

Still, there is a risk, a qualitative risk, one for which I cannot give statistics. All I have is my years of experience as a geriatrician. This is what I bring to the table as I face down the legions of pharmacologists and pharmacists and epidemiologists, medical scientists, smiling, attractive salespersons from Big Pharma, Medicare and Medicaid regulators, chart auditors and quality monitors, and, of course, lawyers, any of whom might be critical of my judgment at a given point in time. All are my allies when things go well; they quickly become my inquisitors when things do not.

There is one major difference between us, however, a difference that separates us now and always: I am the one with the patient before me, a patient—my father or perhaps your mother—who is paranoid or delusional or abusive and in danger of injuring himself or a dedicated caregiver. I am the one you trust, for the moment, to try something, anything, to ameliorate the situation, relieve the tension and the strain and the heartache, the one here now to help diminish the suffering of the old, old man before me and the members of his family. I am the one who must give the order, write the prescription, and face the consequences, for good or ill, of my judgment and my action.

Sometimes, before I reach for a medication, before my father's agitation has risen beyond what he and my family can bear, I put on Sinatra. Or Glenn Miller or Tony Bennett. If I'm lucky that day, my father begins to hum, he taps his foot. Lyrics come, a few at a time: *It was a very good year . . . Pennsylvania 6-5-0-0-0 . . . I left my heart . . .* Sometimes he even tries to whistle along with the melody, but his sagging cheeks and weak facial muscles render him powerless to make a sound. He blows dry, dissonant air.

One afternoon I stop by and he keeps saying over and over in a singsong voice, *I beg your pardon da da da . . . I beg your pardon . . .* Why has my father latched on to this melody?

The next day Yolanda brings him a CD of the complete song, and when I next drop by he is singing the whole first line: *I beg your pardon, I never promised you a rose garden.* I sing along with him.

My mother, sitting in her recliner listening, says, "You never promised me a rock garden, either!"

My father starts laughing, a real guffaw. "You never had much of a sense of humor," he says to her. "But Frances, that was a funny one you just made!"

She chuckles, but I'm not sure she meant to be funny.

Just before my parents' sixtieth wedding anniversary, I find the bottle of risperidone, cut a bunch of the pills in half, and bring my father one of these bisected tablets and a cool glass of his nutritional drink.

"Here, Dad, take this. I think it will make you feel better."

His eyes, still wild, stare at me. "What's this for?"

"Dad, you've got *shpilkes,*" I say. I use this Yiddish word, retrieved somehow from my own memory, because my father has lately been interspersing his speech with snippets of this language, his mother's tongue—the *mamaloschen*—the first words he ever heard, and therefore the last ones to abandon him.

He smiles. "*Az ich haben shpilkes,*" he says. And he swallows the pill. "For the *shpilkes,*" my mother and Yolanda tell him when it is time for the next dose. Before long he is back to his usual demented self, his pleasant self. This time I have made the right decision.

It's time for the sixtieth anniversary brunch. My wife brings a dozen yellow roses and arranges the table. She knows it is the dining set that Grandma Bessie bought my mother and that my family uses it only for special occasions. My brother stops at the grocery store for a side of sliced, smoked salmon, some cream cheese, a few tomatoes, and a red onion. I rise early that morning, drive over to the bagel bakery, and pick up a dozen—onion, poppyseed, and sesame—just out of the oven.

Those of us who love my parents assemble in the brick one-story home where they have lived since first coming to Texas. It is a small gathering. My parents' siblings are long gone, save my father's lone surviving sister, in her mid-nineties and in bad shape herself, a half continent away in Baltimore. Family-oriented to the point of insularity, my parents have made no close friends in all the years they have lived in San Antonio.

Most elders, as they age, find their social connections narrowing: Their kids move away, their brothers and sisters and close friends pass on. As their world implodes, many withdraw further into themselves and this dearth of social contacts only accelerates the decline in cognitive skills. It is a mean cycle, one I try to alter in my patients when I recognize that they are caught up in it. I query them about activities at their church, help them find senior centers, talk to them about volunteer opportunities at the hospital or the library. Over the years,

I have had much more success with the folks in my practice than with my own parents.

So here we are: Lee and I, my brother, his wife Gaye and their son, Adam—my father's only grandson. My daughter Betsy is here and, of course, my parents' devoted health aide, Yolanda. Yolanda is the one who holds everything together in my parents' household and no family celebration is complete without her.

Everything is ready and I wheel my father into the living room.

"What's the fuss about?" he asks as he enters, seeing all these faces he recognizes but cannot place. For a moment he is frightened. Something must have happened: Perhaps someone has died and now he will hear the terrible news.

"Dad," I say, speaking into his good ear, "today is a special day. You and Mom have been married for sixty years."

He searches for my mother's face in the small crowd around him.

"Really? Is that true, Mom?"

"Of course it's true," she says. "Do you think we made this up?"

"It sure doesn't seem like sixty years," he says.

"It seems like a hundred to me," she says. We, the assembled family, laugh nervously.

My brother leans in and asks our father, "So what do you think about all this?"

"I just want to say that I love Mom more today than I ever have." He reaches for her hand, but she doesn't take it. I want to believe that because of her terrible eyesight she can't see this gesture, but I'm not so sure. We all applaud my father's words.

I push him up to the dining room table, festive with cards. He picks out one. "Did you see these, Mom?" he says.

"I can't read them," she answers.

He begins to read to her. They remind him again that it is their anniversary.

"Have we really been married sixty years?" he asks her.

"Every bit of it," she says.

"I hope you know I love you."

"I know," she answers.

"And she loves you, too, Dad," I say.

"Of course she loves me. She's our Mom. She's gotta love all of us," he says.

After the party, after we have cleaned up, the guests have gone home, and I have put my father back to bed, I find my mother sitting on the couch, sobbing softly.

"What is it, Mom? What's the matter?"

"I'm just tired. It's been a long day."

"Mom, it's only early afternoon."

"You know what I mean," she says. And I do. My father's dementia has been progressing now for almost six years. He is getting worse. My mother, like so many spousal caregivers, is ground down, exhausted. My father demands her attention unless he is asleep; she is constantly worried that he is not eating, fearful that he's going to fall, anxious over what will happen next. Most nights he wakes her at least once, maybe more. She has not gotten away on her own now in almost two years.

"Mom, why don't we make plans for you to visit Rita and Buddy in Baltimore for a week or so? It would give you a boost."

"Your father gets worse when I'm not around," she says. And this is true. The last time she went away my brother and I stayed with him, alternated days and nights, back and forth. Our father constantly paced through the house, first to the front door, then to the back, looking for her: "When's Mom coming home? Did something happen? Are you telling me the truth?"

Over and over we explained, told him where she was, called her on the phone so he could hear her voice. "I really miss you, Mom," he said. "When are you coming home to me?"

"Dad," we told him a hundred times, "Mom's in Baltimore visiting Rita and Buddy. She's coming back soon." In the end I resorted to the risperidone. My brother and I were exhausted by the time our mother got home. And she is with him twenty-four/seven. Family caregivers—mostly spouses—give their all, and their high mortality rates (wives often precede their demented or sick husbands to the grave) prove just how grueling this job is.

I take my mother's hand in mine, put my face right up to hers so she can see in my eyes that I mean what I am about to say.

"Mom, listen to me. I know we promised ourselves that we wouldn't put Dad in a dementia unit. But maybe the time has come. He's near the end. You must know this. Mom—it's *you* Mike and I are now most worried about."

Her answer comes without hesitation. "No," she says. "I can't do that. I won't do that."

And then she starts to cry again. I hold her in my arms.

"He's so ugly to me sometimes. He says such terrible things. Especially when you aren't here . . ."

I don't have to ask her what he says. I have heard and I have not forgotten.

"Mom, please try to understand. He's tortured because he's lost himself. Most of the good memories are gone and he's left with distorted ones. You know he's always been a little paranoid about certain things. In his state, these bad memories and feelings take over and he can't control himself. I could increase his medications . . ."

"No," she says. "It settles him down but only confuses him more . . ."

We sit together on the couch for a while. Her mascara, which she has difficulty applying, has run all over her face. I hand her some tissues.

"You know that when Dad says he loves you, he means it, don't you?"

"I think he gets me confused with his own mother," she says.

"Not all the time. I know he loves you. And even though you have a hard time saying it because you're tired and frustrated, I know you love him. He wouldn't be here in this house today if you didn't. And I want to tell you how much I love you—admire you—for this tremendous sacrifice you're making. But if you ever decide enough is enough, I'll find him a place right away."

My mother doesn't answer me. She hears me, has been bolstered by my words. And I have never loved her more than at this moment. I can never make up to her what she has endured—until it is my time to care for her as she has for him.

That time is coming soon.

TWENTY-THREE

As my father's dementia worsens, he is eating less and less. My mother prepares all the foods he used to love: roasted chicken and potatoes with lima beans, cheese blintzes, pot roasts, noodle *kugels*—even his all-time favorite unhealthy meal, kosher hot dogs and baked beans. She leaves the concoction simmering in the pot until the whole house smells like a deli—anything that might stimulate his appetite, entice him to eat. She helps him into the kitchen, settles him into his chair at the table, cuts up his food and sits by his side. She waits for him to say, "I'd like some more." Instead, he pushes his plate away and says, "I'm just not hungry."

At his prime my father was 5 feet 8 inches tall, 175 pounds. Now he is barely over 5 feet and weighs less than 120. He is a parched blade of grass teetering in the wind.

My mother is frantic. "Why won't he eat?" she asks me. "If he doesn't eat, he'll die!"

There are many reasons why someone like my father won't eat.

I thought perhaps he was depressed. When we took him in to see Dr. Galan, we talked about it again. It's natural that my father might be depressed given his current diminished state. We tried different antidepressants. One made him sleep twenty hours a day; on another he paced back and forth between the living room and his bedroom as if he was searching for his lost self. His appetite did not improve.

It must be one of his heart medications, I thought. I changed my father's medications, one at a time. He still wouldn't eat.

I considered appetite stimulants—there are a few on the market— but Dr. Galan was rightly concerned about the potential for excessive heart stimulation and fluid retention and considered these drugs too risky for my father.

He must have an underlying disease, I thought. Something undiagnosed, something terrible, perhaps a colon cancer eating away at his insides. Maybe we should do a colonoscopy, a CAT scan? I knew he was way past the time for aggressive diagnostic evaluations, but I talked to Dr. Galan about it anyway. "What would we do," he said to me, "if we found a colon cancer? You know he couldn't stand an operation or chemotherapy." Of course. But I'm trying to be his son, not his doctor. And anyway, as Dr. Galan astutely noted, his deterioration has been going on for so many years now that if he had a malignant disease he would have been dead long ago.

In 1977 I'd been out in the world of private medical practice for less than a year. In those days before the advent of managed care, before insurance companies directed the flow of patients by contract, one had to build a medical practice one patient at a time. And that was what I was doing one early morning—taking an emergency room consultative call in my hospital. I was heading down the corridor toward the doctor's parking lot when I heard my name echoing over the hospital's paging system.

It was now 2 A.M. I was tired. Two hours before, I'd admitted an elderly man with chest pain, had done all I could for the time being, and was longing to get a few hours of sleep. In six hours I was due back in my office.

I picked up the page.

"Dr. Winakur, this is Dr. Reynolds . . . I'd like you to consult on a patient of mine tonight."

I barely knew Dr. Reynolds—he was a clinical professor of family medicine at the medical school. I had nodded to him in the hospital elevator just two hours ago. Now he was asking for my help. I was tired but flattered.

"Tell me about the patient," I said.

"Mr. Malik is a seventy-eight-year-old man I admitted yesterday with pneumonia. He was improved earlier today. His daughter— she's a bit of an hysteric—asked me to come see him tonight, said he was more short of breath. I did come in for a quick look, and the old man seemed the same to me. I tried to reassure the daughter, but she just called me again through the exchange and insisted on another opinion. I saw you in the hospital earlier. Glad you're still there . . ."

Even then, green as I was in this new world of private practice, I saw all the red flags waving me away from this case: a seasoned doctor calling on me—a neophyte—to help; a family practitioner calling upon a general internist rather than a specialist in cardiology or pulmonary disease; a family member, described as an "hysteric," who has just called her father's doctor twice in the middle of the night. All my instincts for self-preservation told me to decline, to make up an excuse. But I was already worried about this man I had never met.

"Where is he?" I asked.

I found Mr. Malik in a darkened, semiprivate room. His daughter, Helen, hovered over him. Her graying hair was pulled into a tight bun, not a strand out of place. She didn't acknowledge my presence immediately. From the foot of the bed I could see that Mr. Malik's breathing was rapid and shallow and that his skin was bathed in sweat.

I introduced myself.

"Oh, thank God you're here, Doctor. Reynolds is worthless! . . . Two hours ago he stood in this room and said Daddy would be fine in the morning. He didn't even bother to examine him!"

I eased my way past her and let down the bed rail. I reached for Mr. Malik's hand. He was awake and alert but too breathless to talk to me. He nodded in answer to the questions I asked. His pulse was fast and irregular, his lips blue-gray, and his neck veins distended. I listened with my stethoscope to his heart and chest, heard the sounds of air bubbling through drowning lung. Mr. Malik might have had pneumonia when he was admitted, but now he had an abnormal heart rhythm—atrial fibrillation—and his pump was failing, his lungs filling up with fluid. I pressed the nurse call button, asked for the RN on duty, and within moments had arranged for oxygen, diuretics, digitalis, a transfer to intensive care.

I explained to Mr. Malik and his daughter what I thought was wrong and how I intended to remedy the situation. I informed them that I would let Dr. Reynolds know what I had found and what I planned to do, so that he would be up to speed in the morning when he made rounds.

"Oh, no," Helen said. "You're Daddy's doctor now. I'll call Reynolds right now and tell him."

"No. I'll talk with him about this myself." I knew Reynolds would be happy to hear that his services were no longer needed here.

A few hours passed. I hung around the hospital, kept checking on my sick patient. By 5 A.M. Mr. Malik was breathing normally, his pulse rate had slowed nicely, his lips were pink, his skin warm and dry. Helen would not leave her father's side.

"Thank you so much, Doctor. I know you saved my daddy's life tonight. I am so grateful that you came in to see him . . ."

"This is my job," I said.

And I meant it. What I did for Mr. Malik *was* my job, all in a day's work. My medical school professors considered this "garden-variety" medicine. "How many times can you treat congestive heart failure before you get bored with it?" one of them once said to me. This was not cutting edge; this was not high powered, would never lead to a citation in the *New England Journal of Medicine*.

No, I am never bored, but I have been forever anxious. I have been vigilant because I know I am not perfect and because I know that even the most routine case can take an unexpected turn. Thousands of people have come to me with complaints and symptoms, abnormal tests and X-ray results. Every one of them has a unique story; many are puzzles. Despite the fact that I am always anticipating, always worrying, I never expected how Mr. Malik's case would end. Thirty years later I am still haunted by it.

Within two days Mr. Malik was back in a semiprivate room and walking in the halls. Within a week he was stable on just a few medications. He said, "I'll be fine, now, Doctor, if I can just get Helen to leave me alone!" All of us—Helen included—had a good laugh over this.

Helen heaped praise on me every time I made my rounds. I was the best doctor in the world, she said. She was going to change doctors and come to me herself. She was going to tell all her friends about me.

Mr. Malik went home. Helen brought him to my office regularly for his follow-up visits. We got to know each other. He was a good man, a compliant patient with an educated and concerned daughter who constantly looked over his shoulder, and mine.

One night I was called to the emergency room. Mr. Malik had just been brought in by ambulance. I dressed quickly in the dark and rushed to the hospital. I found Mr. Malik on a gurney, waiting in the hallway. He was hard to arouse and the right side of his face drooped. His right arm and leg were paralyzed. A brain scan showed a large stroke in his left cerebral hemisphere.

I sought Helen out in the family waiting room. She was crying.

"Helen, your father's had a big stroke . . ."

"How could this happen? He was doing so well . . ."

"He may have thrown an embolism, a blood clot, from his heart. Or he may have had a stroke from hardening of the arteries . . ."

"Do everything you can, Doctor," Helen said. "You brought him through last time. I know you can do it again . . ."

"This is different," I said. "I'm afraid his brain damage will be severe. He won't be able to speak and may not be able to swallow . . ."

"Just do everything you can. I have faith in you."

Thus began a long siege. Mr. Malik's stroke was a massive one. That night he developed atrial fibrillation again; for a few days he needed a mechanical ventilator to breathe. At one point I had to shock his heart with an external defibrillator in an unsuccessful attempt to normalize his heart rhythm. Then he needed a pacemaker. Although Helen believed she understood her father's grunts and gestures, he was never able to communicate with me again.

I tried to feed Mr. Malik, but he choked on liquids.

"Helen, your father is having trouble swallowing as a result of his stroke," I said. "If we're going to give him every chance, I should insert a feeding tube."

"Will that be hard on him?"

"It can be uncomfortable when I thread the tube through his nose and down his esophagus into his stomach. But it's not dangerous, really."

"Then do it, " Helen said.

"He may never regain his ability to swallow. Then he'll be dependent on the tube feedings to keep him alive. I want you to think about that."

"Just do it, Doctor," she said.

Mr. Malik had left no Advance Directive. Helen wanted me to do everything in my power to keep her father alive. He had two bouts of pneumonia and a urinary tract infection that spread into his bloodstream. The nurses were turning him every two hours to prevent bedsores. Each time Mr. Malik was near death, I brought him back from the brink. Helen was aging before my eyes. Her father had now been in the hospital more than a month.

One evening, as Mr. Malik was recovering from his second bout of pneumonia, I said to Helen: "If he gets pneumonia again perhaps we shouldn't treat it . . ."

"Are you giving up on my father?" Her eyes, ringed by exhaustion, were suddenly lit with fury.

"Of course not. I'm just trying to be realistic about his chances.

He's not going to recover to any significant degree and you are under a terrible strain . . ."

"I'm fine," she said. "Just don't give up on Daddy. I'll never forgive you if you do."

I ran into Dr. Reynolds as I was leaving the hospital that night. I had had no further dealings with him since taking over Mr. Malik's case, but he stopped me in the corridor.

"I see old Malik is back in the hospital," he said to me. "So far I've managed to avoid his daughter."

"He's in bad shape," I said. "Big stroke, lots of complications . . ."

"Well, you're the best man for the job."

"Right," I said, and continued past him to the parking lot.

Mr. Malik was my patient more than thirty years ago, but cases like his occur every day in our hospitals. Elderly patients with devastating illnesses are being kept alive by extraordinary means at the end of their lives. The emotional toll on families is enormous and, of course, the financial cost to society is huge. End-of-life medical care is 27 percent of the Medicare budget, 10 to 12 percent of total health care spending in our country.

My father is alive now only because he drinks four to five cans of a liquid nutritional supplement every day. He will look at the glass in his hand and say, "What am I supposed to do with this?"

"Drink it!" my mother says, and he does. Each can has 250 calories and an assortment of everything he needs to keep him going day to day. I am grateful for this supplement, but is it a "medical intervention"? My father can sit at the table, pick up the glass filled by my mother, lift it to his lips, and drink it, one swallow after the other. Surely, to him, this is no different than drinking a milkshake.

During my residency years it was implicit that my job was to make a correct diagnosis and then to keep my patient alive using whatever means I had. Early in my career the technology, though limited compared to what is available today, included antibiotics and respirators and pacemakers and nasogastric feeding tubes.

In 1975 twenty-one-year-old Karen Ann Quinlan stopped breathing after a night of drinking. At the hospital a bottle of Valium was found in her purse. She was kept alive by a mechanical respirator but remained in a persistent vegetative state, the same kind of wakeful, coma-like condition that Terry Schiavo suffered years later and that was the focus of so much debate in 2005. Karen also required the insertion of a feeding tube in order to continue receiving nutrition. The Quinlan family agonized for months but finally accepted the fact that Karen would almost certainly never regain consciousness. They decided to remove the ventilator that kept her alive.

In 1975—I was in the midst of my internal medicine residency training—the American Medical Association took the position that withdrawal of a respirator from a patient who required one was a form of euthanasia, tantamount to murder. In those days many patients, often elderly and with terminal diseases, were kept alive for long periods of time on ventilators. These patients were heavily sedated, fed through tubes, and unable to interact with their families.

The Quinlan family went to court to remove their daughter from the machine. It was a protracted battle. In 1976 the New Jersey Supreme Court ruled unanimously that the implied right to privacy in our Constitution allows the family of a dying, incompetent patient to withdraw life support. Still, Karen's doctors couldn't bring themselves to switch off the machine. For several weeks they weaned her slowly off the ventilator in the hope that she would breathe on her own. Eventually Karen was able to breathe without the device, but she was still fed through a tube. It was not until 1986, *ten years* after being taken off the respirator, that Karen died of pneumonia.

In 1977 I had managed to keep Mr. Malik alive. He had been on a ventilator only briefly and he was now breathing on his own, but he was not making much progress recovering from his stroke. He was bed-bound, incontinent, unable to speak. I doubted he could understand what was being said to him, but his daughter insisted that he could. This is a scenario played out thousands of times a year: disagreements and misunderstandings between medical professionals and families over just how much a seriously ill patient—particularly one with a stroke—understands. Treading the line between hope and despair with family members is emotionally wrenching and requires much patience, but at some point, when objective recovery is not occurring, the physician must guide the family as other crises in care arise.

Each time Mr. Malik had a life-threatening complication I fought back. My patient, after being in the hospital for almost six weeks, had achieved what doctors resignedly call "maximum hospital benefit." It was time to transfer Mr. Malik to a long-term custodial nursing home. At this point he was being kept alive by good nursing, a few pills crushed and delivered through his nasogastric tube, and, of course, the regular injection of a liquid feeding solution through this same tube at intervals throughout the day.

Supplying supplemental nutrition to a patient like my father seems such a natural thing to do. We each must have a certain number of calories every day to run our body's metabolic machinery and stoke our pumping hearts, a few essential vitamins, minerals, and amino acids to manufacture and repair our myriad enzyme and organ systems and maintain our muscle mass.

Yet I know that there may come a time when my father will be unable to drink his supplement under his own power, a time when, like Mr. Malik, the complicated interplay between the nerves and muscles of swallowing fail due to a stroke or advanced neurological deterioration. Or perhaps one day he will refuse to pick up the glass and follow my mother's command to drink. Then what will we do?

A similar liquid supplement was being pushed down Mr. Malik's feeding tube every few hours. He could not refuse it. He could not taste it. He continued to choke on his own saliva. In 1977 I did not consider feeding my patients via a nasogastric tube a "medical intervention." The nurses considered this part of their normal nursing duties; to all of us then, not feeding a swallowing-impaired patient by tube was tantamount to starving that patient. Then, in 1983, the case of Nancy Cruzan began to play out in the courts.

Nancy Cruzan was a young woman who had been reduced to a persistent vegetative state after sustaining a severe head injury in an automobile accident. She resided in a state-supported home in Missouri (at an annual cost then to taxpayers of about $150,000), and only good nursing care and a feeding tube kept her alive. After seven years Nancy's family asked her caregivers to discontinue her nasogastric tube feedings. The doctors and nurses could not countenance this; they did not perceive her feeding tube as a medical intervention, as Karen Quinlan's mechanical ventilator had been. They believed they were providing Nancy with basic nursing care.

The Cruzan case went to the U.S. Supreme Court and the ruling there, which did not come until 1990, was sweeping. First, the Court recognized the right of a *competent* patient to refuse life-saving medical treatment. The Court also found that a feeding tube is as much a "medical intervention" as a mechanical ventilator, and thus, withdrawing tube feedings was no different from deciding to turn off a breathing machine. Removing such a tube from an *incompetent* patient could be done, although the Court left it to each state to set the standard necessary to make such a judgment. In Missouri, Nancy's home state, the standard of evidence was "clear and convincing"—in general requiring an Advance Directive or Durable Power of Attorney— although enough people who were not family members and knew of Nancy's wishes eventually came forward to convince a lower court that her case met this evidentiary standard. In December 1990 Nancy's physician legally removed her feeding tube. She soon died.

When I was a young internist and Mr. Malik's doctor, I had no Supreme Court precedents to guide me, just my gut instincts and the main tenet of the Hippocratic oath: *First do no harm.* So when I discharged Mr. Malik from the hospital to a long-term-care nursing facility my orders included detailed instructions for his nasogastric feedings. I visited Mr. Malik monthly or whenever Helen thought there was a problem that required my immediate attention, which was often. Helen looked over the shoulders of her father's nursing-home caregivers just as she had done in the hospital. She was a tough woman, no doubt, but as a doctor dedicated to caring for the most vulnerable among us, I appreciated her commitment to her father.

Despite Helen's fierce love and devotion, despite physical therapy, respiratory therapy, excellent nursing care, and supplemental nutrition, Mr. Malik suffered the ravages of his age, of being bed-bound, mute, and half-paralyzed, of being unable to swallow, of requiring a long-term bladder catheter. He developed muscle-wasting, skin tears, bedsores, recurrent infections; underwent emergency room transfers and hospital readmissions, multiple needle sticks, intravenous infusions, courses of antibiotics, the colonization of his body with resistant germs. I wanted to let him go, to let nature take its course. At every juncture Helen and I talked about this being the "last time" we would treat his pneumonia, the "last time" we would transfer him to the hospital. But she would not relent—until the day she'd had enough.

She called me to his nursing home bedside; he had been there about six months. He no longer responded to any stimulus other than pain.

"Doctor, I want you to pull out his feeding tube. Now," she said.

For a moment I was speechless. I nodded toward the hallway. I doubted Mr. Malik understood a word that was being spoken, but I could not be certain. Helen followed me out into the corridor.

"Helen, I can't do that," I said. "The nursing staff will be up in arms. What you're asking me to do is tantamount to euthanasia."

"He has suffered enough. I will not countenance this another minute," she said. Her face was as rigid as the tile floor. The fury— as well as the unrealistic hope—I had once seen in her eyes was gone.

"Helen, it's inevitable that your father will get another infection—pneumonia or another urinary tract infection. Let's decide here and now that when the time comes we won't treat it, that we'll just keep him comfortable . . ."

"I want that tube out now, Doctor, or you're off Daddy's case!"

I dug in my heels, but I felt terrible as I heard my own words.

"I'm sorry, but I can't."

"Then, good-bye, Doctor."

I walked the long corridor to the nurse's station and sat down. I picked up Mr. Malik's heavy chart. I turned to the "Physician Progress Notes" section and I recorded what had just transpired. It felt as if someone else's hand was making that entry. I made it clear that I remained Mr. Malik's doctor until Helen could find someone to replace me, if she could.

I didn't sleep that night. After all I had tried to do for Mr. Malik—had done for him—I felt as if I were now abandoning him. Yes, I was angry with Helen. She was a difficult and obstinate woman, perhaps even a bit mad. But I believed—perhaps naïvely so then—that it was my responsibility to negotiate the often difficult dynamics of the doctor-patient-family relationship. This was part of my job, and I had failed.

Mr. Malik didn't live much longer. He died from complications of an untreated pneumonia under someone else's care. A week or so after she dismissed me as her father's doctor and after she was unable, in 1977, to find a physician who would pull out her father's feeding tube, I received a letter from Helen. Since I no longer have this note I must paraphrase it, but after all these years its essence remains vivid in my memory: "I can only hope," she wrote, "that your own father suffers a slow and lingering death like the one you have forced mine to endure."

I don't believe in curses or omens. Yes, my father is dying slowly by degrees. And yes—though he denies it—at times he is suffering. But what about Mr. Malik? What about Karen Quinlan and Nancy Cruzan or Terry Schiavo? Who is suffering in cases like this, cases—

unlike my father's—where patients are comatose or in persistent vegetative states?

The families are suffering. These people watch a loved one diminish, retreat from life into a shell, where the withered self no longer communicates or responds in any meaningful way. Doctors can almost always relieve pain; morphine has been around a long time. But most of us fail to treat suffering, the existential morass of losses before actual death—of independence, mutually supportive companionship, of selfhood. And fear of the unknown. We often fail our patients and their families because we avoid their gaze and their hard questions, apprehensive over what we ourselves might see in their eyes.

When I refused to acknowledge Helen's suffering, I appeared callous and unempathic to her. I was angry with Helen for not appreciating all the excellent medical care I had given her father, for saving his life so many times. She was demanding and irrational. She didn't appreciate my ethical predicament. She didn't care a whit that I, too, was exhausted and had many other patients to care for besides her father—nor should she have. But she was the one who was suffering and I failed her.

Many years have passed since I was Mr. Malik's doctor. The legal answers to the difficult decisions surrounding feeding tubes are clearer. This is not to say that these decisions are easy—they never are. But now I can come to a family in the midst of a crisis and say: "Let us put in a feeding tube for a period of time. Let's give your mother every chance now. If we find in a few days or a few weeks that the long-range outcome is grim, well, we can talk about these tube feedings again, decide if we want to continue them or not."

I do not believe in euthanasia. Still, in fitful sleep, I have dreamed of a time when I go to my father's bed, syringe in hand, and say, "I love you, Dad," and "Good-bye, Dad" as I push the drugs into his bloodstream. But I know that I could never do this to my father or to anyone like

him. I am too deeply steeped in the tradition of medicine, too rooted
in the art of healing.

I have had many years to reflect on Helen's letter to me. I wish I
had taken her away from the darkened room in which her father had
been dying for so many months. Maybe we would have walked into
the courtyard of the nursing home and sat down together at one of
the tables under a canvas umbrella, just out of the bright sun, where I
could look into her face, into those eyes that were once so full of love
and rage in defense of her father.

"Helen," I should have said, "I know you are sad and angry and
frustrated over what has happened to your father. I see how much
you are suffering with the burden of his care and the decisions you
feel you must make. How much you miss him, the man he was. I
know you have reached the end of your rope; I see how much you
just want it to be over. But I promise you that it will be over soon. I
promise you that he is not in pain and that I honestly do not believe
he is suffering now. And I promise that as long as I am his doctor he
will not suffer and that I will do nothing more to prolong his life.
His time is near and I will be here for you and for him when that
time comes."

Had I taken the time to say these few sentences, had I the training
or the wisdom at that stage of my career, I believe that Mr. Malik's
death would have occurred on my watch. I would have filled out and
signed his death certificate. This is what a physician in the true and full
sense of the word can do.

There are those who will say, even today, that to discontinue
a medical intervention that is keeping someone alive—turning off a
ventilator or pulling out a feeding tube—is tantamount to murder.
To them I say that caring for Mr. Malik and the many like him on
whom I have laid my hands through the years has made me aware
of the acute suffering of loved ones during the course of my patients' illnesses and declines. I believe that it is my responsibility to
reduce, as much as possible, unneeded suffering in the small world
that is my patients' and their families'. Sometimes it is most merciful

to relieve that suffering by finally having the courage to switch off
the lights and say good-bye.

One day my father will no longer drink his supplement. He will
have forgotten how to lift a glass to his lips and swallow. Even with
prompting he will be unable to do this. Or perhaps he will no longer
have the will to live. He will lie in his bed, close his eyes and wait.
The chocolate liquid will remain in a glass on the kitchen table. My
mother, who nourished her two sons to adulthood, will wring her
hands. My brother will ask me, a doctor of the oldest old, about a
feeding tube. I will explain to him that there is no reliable medical
data supporting the use of tube feedings in demented patients like
our father. That despite our best intentions, much harm may accrue.

I will resist with all my might the impulse to deliver this fluid to
my father by any route other than through his own mouth. I will sit
him up in bed or in a chair. I will moisten his lips, drip in supplement
by straw or by spoon. I will talk to him, cajole him; be stalwart when
he coughs or chokes, patient when he refuses. I will come back later
and try again. Each time I leave I will say my final good-bye to him.
And on each of those days I will hope that the last one comes soon.

TWENTY-FOUR

In recent months my father has been wandering in the night. He cannot go very far. He turns on his bedroom light, fumbles for his glasses, and puts them on. He searches for his slippers but they are not there because we have hidden them. He drags one leg now and slippers only impede his progress, make it more likely that he will fall.

The walker waits by his bedside and he will hoist himself up into it and search the house for my mother, who is asleep in the next room. He turns on every light—hallway, living room, dining room, kitchen. The exterior doors are dead-bolted and my mother keeps the key with her at all times.

My father stands at the threshold of her bedroom and peers in at the person asleep there. He is not sure who it is. He comes over for a closer look. Sometimes she feigns sleep in the hope that he will return to his own bed.

But now he recognizes her. "Can I get you something, sweetheart?"

"Leonard, please let me sleep! I'm so tired. Go back to your room."

"I'm sorry I woke you, sweetheart," he says. Yes, it is his wife; she is here in the house with him. Now he can rest. He shuffles back down the hall, pushing his walker before him, back to his room, turns off the bedside light, eventually falls back to sleep. Then, once again, my mother gets up and turns off all the lights he has left on.

In the last few months he is worse at night. He comes into her room and sits on her bed. Often he is crying. "Please tell me who I am," he pleads. "I don't know who I am . . ."

My mother is exhausted. Again my brother and I hire someone to sit with him at night, but this strange person serves only to fuel our father's confusion and paranoia. We have to let her go after the first week.

"Please tell me who I am . . ." he says.

My mother moves over in her bed. "Lie down next to me. It's cold. Get under the covers."

"Are you sure you want me to?" he asks.

"Get under, Len. Try to go back to sleep."

"Is my mother still living?"

"She's been dead a long time. You know that."

"What about Frank?"

"Frank died forty years ago."

By now my father is weeping. He asks about Hilda and Mary and Arthur and Sylvia. They are all gone, save Sylvia. Every night my mother buries my father's family and he mourns anew.

"Mom," I beg, when she relates these nightly episodes, "can't you just say everyone is fine back in Baltimore. It's cruel to tell him the truth."

"I can't lie to him," she says.

"Why not? It's a helpful lie, a good lie."

"I just can't lie to your father. Maybe there's something else he can take . . ."

"Dr. Galan and I have tried everything."

"I know, I know," she says.

But again, after consultation with his doctor, I try something else. My father sleeps better for a few nights, but then begins to have a hard time waking up in the mornings.

"He's sleeping all the time," my mother complains on the phone. "He won't eat, not even the chocolate drink . . ."

I get out the pill cutter. I halve pills. I quarter them. They turn to powder. I mix them in applesauce. I dilute to homeopathic doses.

"He's keeping me up at night again," she says. "He's wandering all over the house, turning on the lights. Last night he came in and told me there were men in his room. I opened his closet door to show him no one was there. Finally he went to sleep."

For decades now I have been issuing warnings to my patients and their families. I tell them to lose weight or expect a heart attack, take their blood pressure medications or have a stroke, stop smoking or get cancer, pull up the throw rugs or fall. And on and on. Some people listen, change their lives and sometimes even their medical outcomes. Most listen only sometimes, many not at all. I am their doctor, come what may. I listen, I cajole, I explain, I educate. In this I am not alone. There are thousands and thousands of patient, empathic doctors out there.

But I am not my father's doctor; I am his son. It is true he is much diminished from the man I once knew; yet in some essential way, he is still my father. And even though he is demented, even though I have his power of attorney, even though I am his legally appointed surrogate health-care decision maker, I am only one member of my family. I do not want the weight of every decision to rest on my shoulders as long as my mother is competent and my brother continues to play an active role. But I am the doctor in the family; I have special knowledge, a learned patience, observational skills honed over decades.

And still the nights are bad. My father is only getting worse.

———

Last year I got one of those calls that come every so often from a medical malpractice attorney. An elderly man, Mr. Travis Johnson, with Parkinson's disease as well as psychiatric issues, walked out of a hospital in a distant Texas city. He was found a week later, dead, under a railroad trestle some miles away.

"It's an elopement case against the hospital," the attorney says. Such a strange term. It conjures up images of romance, of adventure; a maverick act, of taking the road less traveled. I'd never been involved in an elopement case before. A lot of publicity surrounded this one: grisly newspaper articles and TV reportage.

Boxes and boxes of records land on my desk, ten years of medical history. Mr. Johnson was a man a decade younger than my father, but unlike him he smoked and drank and used drugs. At heart he was a simple man, a cowboy who spent his youth in far West Texas and longed to return there. He had no close-knit family, no external support system. He had multiple admissions to hospitals, skilled units and long-term-care facilities. A note in his medical chart stated that Mr. Johnson had been depressed—he said once that life was not worth living.

My review of all the records and reports convinced me that Mr. Johnson received excellent medical care. His daughter admitted as much. When he took his medications—he was on five psychoactive drugs—she said he was manageable, but he didn't like the way the drugs made him feel and when he wasn't being supervised he stopped them.

Mr. Johnson was admitted to the hospital that last time because he had once again discontinued his medications and worsened. After just a few days, after a complete re-evaluation by his doctors, after his medications were re-started at reduced dosages, he improved. When last seen in the hospital he was walking the halls, waiting to be picked up by the van coming to take him back to the long-term-care facility where he had lived before.

On the day Mr. Johnson was discharged from the hospital, he dressed himself and put on his calfskin boots. He doffed the white Stetson he always wore. He walked the halls, rounded the nurses' station again and again, smiled and tipped his hat at the staff, waited for the van. And then he disappeared. The nurses quickly realized that Mr. Johnson was missing and carried out an extensive search of the hospital and its immediate environs. They notified the police, but that was the last time anyone saw him alive.

According to the police report, Mr. Johnson was discovered a week later underneath a railroad trestle, his hat and boots neatly arranged beside his body. The report went on to state that Mr. Johnson had probably spent a lot of time there because the dirt had been smoothed and packed; a well-worn trail wound through the underbrush leading down to a small stream. The investigating officer concluded that Travis Johnson had been dead for at most two days from natural causes, not foul play.

In my opinion letter I wrote that Mr. Johnson was functioning—when on his medications and under caring supervision—as an autonomous individual. He was able to make his needs known, sign his own consent forms, state his unhappiness about living in an institutional setting. His depression developed because his medical and psychiatric problems prevented him from doing the things he used to enjoy. Though there may have been times when he needed closer monitoring—and his physicians were aware of this—most of the time he was capable of making his own decisions.

Respect for individual autonomy is the cornerstone of the ethical treatment of patients. The long-term institutionalization of the mentally ill in our society has virtually disappeared as more effective treatment of most psychiatric illnesses has evolved. This speaks to the tantamount importance of allowing autonomously functioning individuals to live as outpatients and make decisions for themselves.

No one can know, I went on to say in my report, what was in the mind of Travis Johnson when he walked out of the hospital that day. We cannot know if he was planning to go home to his daughter or attempting to return to West Texas. He did make a conscious decision to go off by himself, maybe even perhaps to hasten his own death. He did choose a place to hide, to live on his own for several days, just a short walk from a highway where he might have been discovered had he wanted to be found.

Mr. Johnson's death, I concluded, was a tragic one. His leaving the hospital was unforeseen by his three physicians who knew his social, medical, neurological, and psychiatric history and who had the power to write orders for closer observation and even restraints. But they chose not to issue these orders, I believe, because they considered Travis Johnson to be—at that point in time—oriented, nonsuicidal, and with adequate judgment to function autonomously. And without any orders from his doctors to the contrary, the hospital staff treated him as they would any elderly patient with a chronic medical condition. They had no reason to suspect that he would leave the hospital grounds.

The tension in this case, then, is between two conflicting ethical principles—autonomy and beneficence. Mr. Johnson's caregivers wanted to do their best to keep him safe, protect him from danger, even if that danger was from himself; and yet most of the time he was able to function as an autonomous individual.

Dr. Leon Kass, former chairman of the President's Council on Bioethics, has this to say about the treatment of our elderly and this tension between autonomy and beneficence, specifically with regard to Advance Directives:

> [T]his emphasis on autonomy ignores the truth of human interdependence and of our unavoidable need for human presence and care, especially when we can no longer take care of ourselves. The moral emphasis on choosing in advance needs to be replaced with a moral emphasis on caring in the present.

Dr. Kass asks us to re-commit ourselves to serving our loved ones, their disabilities notwithstanding. Instead of putting so much emphasis on legal directives documenting what we will *no longer do* for an incapacitated elder (as important as these instructions are in end-of-life situations), he asks all of us—professional caregivers as well as family—to devote ourselves to the daily welfare of our disabled loved ones.

The Johnson case settled out of court. Over the years I have been designated as an expert witness in a number of other medical mal-practice cases involving the treatment—usually nursing-home care—of an elderly individual. Sometimes the event precipitating the lawsuit is truly egregious and should never have happened. I cannot defend cases like these and I don't. Most of the time, however, the ravages of aging and disease and dementia are to blame for the final outcome. People are going to die when they are in their eighties and nineties and have reached the stage in life when they need long-term custo-dial nursing-home care. If they were not in a nursing home they would die at home or in a hospital. Families sometimes forget this. They are driven by years of anger and guilt (and occasionally greed) which is often misplaced onto the provider of last resort, the nursing home. This is not a defense of substandard hospital or nursing-home care—none of us should tolerate that. But our limited dollars and energies could be much better spent in the care of our elderly rather than in litigation.

When I completed my residency training more than thirty years ago I thought I knew everything I needed to know about the practice of medicine. I passed my Board examinations, confidently set up an of-fice, and with the arrogance of youth believed I was the best-trained, most qualified internist around. Now that I am on the verge of be-coming old myself, I find I am less and less certain about more and more. Perhaps this is wisdom, although of a discomfiting sort.

I am so often wrong about how my patients will die. Not a week goes by that I don't lose someone I have known for years—decades, even. I know the intimate details of her medical and social and family history. I know how much she drinks, how many cigarettes he smokes each day. I have seen her scars, the real and the emotional. I am familiar with his heart sounds, how the edge of his liver feels when I ask him to breathe deeply and the organ rolls down over the tips of my fingers. I have an updated list of each and every diagnosis my patients carry, every drug I prescribe, letters from every consultant to whom I have sent them, reports on every imaging procedure I ever ordered, a chronological sequence of blood and urine test results going back for years. Still, I cannot, most of the time, know when and how my patients will leave this earth.

Mr. Mason, with extensive cancer throughout both lungs, returned to his boyhood home in Mississippi years ago to die. He is still sending me e-mails. Mrs. Freeman, with severe emphysema from cigarettes, lived alone on her ranch in the Hill Country, tending her sheep and her goats until she fell down an abandoned well. Sister Enid changed doctors to see one of my younger associates; she feared I was on the brink of retirement and would not be there for her when she needed me. She died in the blink of an eye from cancer while I still see my patients week after week. Young and vigorous, Mr. Laughton came in one day for his yearly physical. A spot showed up on his chest X-ray that turned out to be a mesothelioma, an aggressive form of cancer related to asbestos exposure. He had never been near this material in his life. I watched as he lost a hundred pounds, failed to respond to any treatment, disintegrated before my eyes. He died, this strong man with small children, by his own hand.

I could go on and on. We never know what life has in store for us; statistics, valid in large groups, devolve to meaningless blather at the level of the individual. My father is one of our nation's oldest old. For three decades he has lived with a badly damaged heart. And then prostate cancer. Conventional wisdom—guided by population studies of mortality rates in large groups—says my father should have died a long time ago. And yet here he is, still alive, lurching from one day into the next.

All his nocturnal activity, all this wandering—how does my father do it? He can barely make it from his bedroom to the commode a few steps away. He leans on walls, the edges of furniture, thresholds, doorways. His body is as bent as an open safety pin. My mother is not getting enough rest. She is a burned-out caregiver; all the studies show that she is at risk for depression, illness, and a shortened life expectancy.

I try again to get her to take a week off, to travel back to Baltimore, visit her cousins.

"I'll stay with him. Mike and I will take turns," I say.

"He'll be frantic if I leave," she says. "He comes looking for me. I'm the only one who can settle him down."

I try to talk to my father. I suspect it is useless, but we sit together on the sagging living room couch one evening before his bedtime.

"Dad, you have to stay in bed all night. Even if you wake up— unless you're in pain or in trouble somehow—you've got to let Mom sleep. Stop waking her up."

"I don't do that. Frances, do I wake you up?"

"Only every night," she says.

"I didn't realize that. I'm sorry, sweetheart . . ." He starts to cry.

"Dad, it's okay. Just try to remember to let Mom sleep, okay?"

"I'm not too happy with myself either, you know," he says through his tears. I am shocked by his ability to comprehend and the lucidity of his words.

"It's okay, Dad. We all know you're doing the best you can . . ."

"I'm an old man now," he says.

The nighttime perambulations continue.

"Mom," I say, "this can't go on. I think it's time for him to go into a dementia unit. I promised myself I would never do it. But I'm concerned about you now more than him . . ."

"No. He's staying right here."

"Something bad is going to happen. He's going to fall in the night and break his hip . . ."

"We'll worry about that when the time comes," she says.

TWENTY-FIVE

On the morning of February twenty-eighth, four days after my parents' sixtieth wedding anniversary, my father elopes. Without his bride. Without his walker. He does not go far.

I am just walking into my office to begin seeing patients for the day. My cell phone rings.

My brother's voice shakes. "I'm at Mom's," he says. "Dad's in the backyard . . . EMS is here . . ."

"EMS?" I ask, stunned. "My God, Michael, don't let them do anything. I'll be right there." I hear wailing in the background.

"I think it's too late," he says.

I find Anna and Alyson, my office manager and my medical assistant. Anna has been with me thirty years, Alyson twenty. They are both stricken, but, as always, they swing into action. "We'll take care of everything here," they assure me as I run out the door.

From my office it's a ten-minute ride to my parents' house. This morning it seems to take an hour. I find myself thinking about my father's early life, about the year 1935, the Great Depression, my father's father already dead nine years. How Dad joined his older sister Mary in the pawnshop, and these two—a sixteen-year-old boy and his twenty-eight-year-old sister—ran this tough business in downtown Baltimore not far from the Bowery.

On the drive to his home where my old, old father now lies in the backyard, my mind is flooded with these stories of his life, stories he had told me over and over again during my boyhood, usually when we were out fishing together, our rented rowboat rocking at anchor on the South River, or the Severn, or in the Kent Narrows. There was something about those times—the salt air, the daylight dawning over the Eastern Shore, the lap of water on the wooden hull, the anticipation—that enabled him to muse without bitterness about who he was, about the person he had become.

. . . I was never much of a student anyway, you know. I never could spell and my handwriting was awful. Arthur, now, he was the smart one and Hilda, too, so they got to finish school and go to college . . . So I was in the pawnshop. I started cleaning up the out-of-pawn items, polishing the jewelry, putting new bands and crystals on the watches if they needed it . . . I got a little salary, bought a car, went on some dates . . . Life was good. Granny was proud of me. I bought her things . . . "I can do this!" I said to myself. My life is going to be okay. And the best part was when I met your mother . . .

The EMS van is parked out front, lights spinning. Emergency medical crews are an indispensable arm of our modern health-care system. There is an EMS substation around the corner from my parents' home. They can be there in two minutes, maybe less.

When the heart stops, brain cells begin to starve from lack of oxygen. They die off in the millions. The first ones to go, the ones in our frontal lobes, store memory and language. This is the locus of cognition, the part of our brain that makes us each uniquely who we are. The last cells to die—within minutes still—are the ones in our lower brain and brain stem, the involuntary, automatic connections that regulate our heartbeats, our breathing and blood pressure, our basic reflexes to withdraw from pain and to gag. The delicate balance— the great danger—is always this: In trying to save the higher functions, we may end up having preserved only the automatic ones. Then what?

How many times did we—my mother, my brother, and I—talk about calling EMS in the event of an emergency?

"Mom," I said again and again, "one day something will happen to Dad. Please, whatever happens, don't call 911! Call me or Mike, but remember, there is no reason anymore to call EMS for Dad."

"I know. I know," she said.

Most people in similar situations panic and dial 911 unless hospice is involved and the families have been coached over and over. Even then there is often guilt that can last a long time: *Maybe we could have saved Mom or Dad . . .*

Families of the oldest old are not aware that in a large study of cardiopulmonary resuscitation (CPR) attempts—182 elderly patients resuscitated in their nursing facilities—not a single one of these heroic acts led to an intact individual leaving the hospital. Resuscitating people like my father is considered a prime example of "futile" care in the elderly. There may be those who say these efforts and expenditures must be made, that it is inhumane to do otherwise. To them I will simply answer that in order to have the resources as a nation to provide a decent level of care to our aging population—for our entire populace—we must try very hard to eliminate each identified example of futile care.

When the emergency medical technicians (EMTs) enter my parents' home, they see an old woman in her pajamas sobbing in the living room, another panicked woman in the backyard bent over a body, doing her best to perform CPR. They do not know that the old, old man on the ground has already lost most of the brain cells they are rushing in to save, that he is dying of a progressive, terminal disease for which there is no cure, that in many ways this man—the father that I still love—left us long ago.

By the time I arrive, my mother sits in the living room, an anguished look on her face. Yolanda, sobbing, kneels by her side and holds her hand. The EMTs are around the dining room table, filling out paperwork. I look at them and they both shake their heads.

I bend down and kiss my mother. For the first time, she looks all of her eighty-two years. "It's over now, Mom," I say.

"Did you see him?" she asks.

"Not yet," I say and start down the hallway to his bedroom. I have always hoped he would die in his own bed, in his sleep. But as a doctor I have learned through the years that there is almost always a great struggle in the end.

One of the EMTs stops me, tugs me gently by the arm. "He's in the backyard," he says.

"Yes. Right. Of course."

My brother is sitting by my father, but he gets up when I step outside. We hug each other.

"Our father's gone," he says.

"He's been gone a long time, Mikey." I am too accustomed to death; I worry that I have become too hardened because of it.

I kneel beside my father and look into his face. His worn and worried expression, his confused demeanor is gone now. I cradle his head in my hands. His skin is blue-gray. I raise his eyelids and peer into dilated, clear pupils. I palpate the bones of his skull, feeling for bruises, looking for matted hair, coagulated blood. There is no sign of injury. I look at his hands, his arms, his legs. I move his hips around in their sockets. His body is not in rigor. I cannot find any evidence of trauma.

"How did he get out here?" I ask my brother.

He points to a seldom-used door from the garage into the backyard. It is ajar. My parents never parked in the garage. Always fearing an intrusion, my father sealed the sliding garage doors at the front of the house with a series of C-clamps. Years ago, when my father was painting in his garage studio—and since there were no windows— he installed an air conditioner into the door that opens onto the backyard and fixed a heavy sliding bolt on the inside to keep it shut and impenetrable from the exterior.

I walk into the garage through the door my father had exited. It is heavy with the weight of the AC unit and groans on its hinges. I close the door behind me and I try to throw the rusted bolt back into place. It takes all my strength. How my father got it open I will never know.

From the garage I walk through another door directly into the kitchen. This door has a keyed dead bolt on it—and my mother's keys are dangling from the lock on the kitchen side of the door. During the day she is constantly running in and out of the garage through this door—to do the laundry or to bring in the cans of my father's nutritional supplement from the storage shelves there. Last night she had forgotten and left the keys in the dead bolt.

The EMTs are finishing up their paperwork.

"What did you find?" I ask.

They are both very professional, these two young men in their blue uniforms. But more important, they are kind and compassionate. I have had only positive encounters with men and women like these over the years.

"He didn't have anything on the heart monitor. Nothing. His temp was ninety-two degrees. We're sorry we couldn't do more . . ."

I am caught off guard by this number. It isn't quite spring in San Antonio; the air temperature that morning was fifty degrees. He couldn't have been outside very long, maybe a couple of hours, maybe less. Still, my father—old, thin, and wasted, with a bad heart, poor circulation, unprotected from the cold—probably died of hypothermia, went to sleep and had a fatal cardiac arrhythmia. Hypothermia is a gentle way to die. After the shivering stops, one just goes to sleep. I cannot help but think: Had my father exposed himself to the early morning chill on purpose?

I walk back over to my mother and sit down on the couch next to her chair. Yolanda still kneels by her side, her hands cradling my mother's.

"Mom," I ask. "What happened?"

"He was all confused last night. Michael knows how bad he was— he was here with him for a while and got him settled down. 'I want to go home,' he kept saying, 'please take me home.' Then Michael called you and you told him to give Dad one of those pills . . ."

Of course I remember: I told my brother to give him another risperidone tablet.

"What about in the night?" I ask her.

"I was worried he wouldn't sleep and I tried to get him to come into my bed. He sleeps better sometimes if he's next to me. But he went into his own room."

"Did he wake you?" I asked.

"He always wakes me. You know how he is. He walks around, turns on all the lights, comes into my room. But he didn't wake me last night. Usually I hear him when he gets up, but I was so exhausted last night . . ."

"What happened this morning?"

"I got up just before nine and went to check on him and he wasn't in his bed. I started looking all over the house. I couldn't find him—'Len,' I'm calling, 'Len'—I was frantic and then Yolanda came and I told her I couldn't find Leonard. She searched everywhere, all the closets. Then she saw him outside on the lawn . . ."

"What about the lights? Were they on?"

"No. He hadn't turned on even one light . . ."

So the day had already dawned when my father eloped into the backyard. He couldn't have been out there very long.

The EMTs are packing up to leave. My father is still outside on the grass, my brother with him.

"Can't we bring him inside?" I say.

"The police will be here to make their report," one of the technicians answers. "I'm sorry," he says.

And then it hits me. My father died at home, outside. It is an unusual circumstance, not a "natural" death. He will be a medical examiner's case.

"Wait," I say. "Perhaps I should talk to the medical examiner. My father has—had—a significant dementia. This was not really unexpected and I'd hate to have him hauled downtown for an autopsy . . ."

"Talk to the investigators when they get here. I'm sorry," he says again.

My brother comes inside just then. His eyes are red and swollen.

"I'll call the funeral home," he says. "Someone should sit with Dad."

I go out into the backyard. My father looks like a small bird lying there in the grass.

I move a plastic lawn chair from the patio close to my father and sit. The sun is warming the day, and even though the bird feeder is empty, the cardinals and titmice and chickadees are flitting back and forth in the bare branches of the big pecan.

The pyracanthas still have plenty of red berries and the mocking-birds and blue jays call from their perches on the back fence as they dart in and out of the bushes. Sitting with my father, watching the birds fly through the yard, hearing the incantatory murmurings of the white-winged doves perched in the branches, I feel some small measure of peace descend upon my family.

I will never know what my father was thinking that morning. I know what I want to believe: It is early light when he arises. He feels strong, young. He leaves his walker behind in the bedroom. He passes by the door of his sleeping wife, peers in at her face. *Let her rest,* he thinks to himself, *she's been under a great strain.* He makes his way slowly into the kitchen and he sits a while at the table, catches his breath. He stares out over the back lawn. The sun is just up and the birds are flitting back and forth in the old pecan. He sees that the feeder is empty and remembers that somewhere out back there is a bin with a tight-fitting lid full of sunflower seeds. He stands up and walks the two steps over to the door that leads into the garage. The key is in the lock; he turns it and the door opens easily. Once inside the garage, he struggles with the rusty bolt on the other door that will let him out into the yard. *This damn thing has always been hard,* he mutters to himself. He pulls and yanks on it with hands strong from supporting himself in his walker. Finally the bolt slides free. The door opens onto a glorious morning. The air is cool, but he is wearing his sweat suit and heavy white socks. The dawn chorus is in full throat and for the first time in years he can hear the trills and tremolos, the sweet risings and fallings of the bird songs he recalls from the backyard of the house on Boarman Avenue.

But he is starting to feel a little cold and he has no stores of fat, no heavy muscle. He wears no jacket, no hat, no shoes. He looks around for the bird feeder and sees the green metal dish sitting on the other side of the patio on the shelves he once built to hold his geraniums and petunias. He starts for it, but his legs—those long skinny legs that carried him swiftly around the high-school track—betray him and he goes down into the grass.

He begins to shiver. He struggles for a while to get up. He can't understand what is so difficult about getting up. He's fallen a thousand times and has always gotten up. He thinks about yelling for his wife, but he doesn't want to wake her. Besides, she will be up soon and see him out here on the lawn and help him up. Probably give him hell, too, for going outside without her.

But it's okay because nothing hurts; he is comfortable in the grass, the sun is rising higher in the sky, the birds are singing in the treetops. He has always been a patient man, survived whatever life held in store. He rolls onto his side. He has stopped shivering now and sleep overtakes him . . .

. . . *Okay, Jerry-boy, this is prime fishin' time . . . keep spooning that chum over the side . . . see how it drifts out behind the boat in the tide? Perfect, a perfect day, a little overcast, not much wind, tide runnin' strong . . . they're out there, I know it . . . somewhere out there in the tide just waiting . . . Now watch how I do it . . . slip the clamsnout onto the hook just like a worm . . . then flip it out into the chum line, that's it, son, just like that . . . Now open your bail and let the tide take your line, feed it out little by little . . . they're out there . . . God I love this . . . What a morning . . . Keep spoonin' out that chum, Jerry-boy . . . feed that line out through your fingers and when it starts to run away like hell, takes off toward the lighthouse, count to three, flip your bail, and set the hook. Hard. Set it hard . . . they're out there. I can feel it. Be patient . . . be patient and you'll hook one . . . and then be ready for the fight of your life . . . Just be patient and your time will come . . .*

TWENTY-SIX

The police arrive.

I review my father's medical history and give them his doctor's phone number. In a short while the medical examiner calls to tell me there will be no further inquiry into his death. Two men from the funeral home pick up his body from the backyard. My brother and I stay with him until the van drives away. We comfort our mother as best we can. "I just keep seeing him out there on the ground," she says.

My brother calls the rabbi, makes all the necessary arrangements. Jews bury their dead within twenty-four hours if at all possible. My parents had bought cemetery plots a few years before, the one solemn acknowledgment of their mortality.

That afternoon, Michael and I drive to the mortuary to make the plans. This means, of course, picking a casket and paying in advance for the burial. This is our first experience at this. We are shepherded into a little room by a salesman who hands us color brochures. It is like buying a car without any joy in the purchase.

Here is what the mortuary will do for my father: Two men pick him up from the yard and put him in the van; they will refrigerate him overnight; a single hearse will drive him to the cemetery; they will erect a small tent over the grave, sheltering half a dozen folding chairs; they will place a mechanism to lower the casket over the hole dug by the cemetery workers. They will provide a "registration booklet" and a package of "thank you for your expression of sympathy" cards at no extra charge.

Then there is, of course, the box.

"Let us pick the casket now," the mortuary man says. My brother and I know what we want—a simple pine box in keeping with the traditions of our religion—and we say so.

"I must insist you view all the caskets," he says. "I wouldn't want you to be disappointed at the cemetery." My brother and I look at each other. Neither of us is in a mood to be rude. The mortuary man shows us into a huge room overflowing with caskets—dark mahoganies, shiny metals, boxes with silk and satin interiors—some priced as high as ten thousand dollars.

We choose the simplest pine box, a few boards nailed together, straw in the bottom, no liner whatsoever, a wooden Star of David glued onto the lid. This purchase alone is almost a thousand dollars. My father could have built it in a couple of hours, using hand tools. All in all, we spend six thousand dollars that day.

I think about all my vulnerable elderly patients, those bereaved widows and widowers, often with no one to protect them from the pitchmen, the not-so-subtle guilt-mongers of the mortuary industry. A shiver runs down my spine.

The day after my father dies, Lee and I drive my mother and Yolanda to the cemetery. There is a heavy silence in the car. I say, "It's so quiet in here, you'd think we were on our way to a funeral!" Yolanda laughs her deep, throaty laugh. Even my mother smiles but then quickly says, "I just keep seeing him in the grass . . ."

"Mom," I say. "You've been a wonderful wife all these years. You have nothing to feel guilty about." I know this is not the end of it.

I am surprised at the crowd. I had a nagging concern that we wouldn't have enough men to bear my father's casket to the grave, that we wouldn't have enough Jewish people—ten—for the requisite prayer *minyen*. I needn't have worried. Many of the ladies my mother had worked with at my office are here, my brother's friends from his shul, my first wife, Leslie, and her mother, my doctor colleagues, lots of my friends, many of them my patients.

Now it is time to bury Dad, to say a few words, chant the Kaddish, lower him into the ground. Jewish graveside services are short and to the point. Being there, under the old live oaks, those stalwart observers, takes me back over four decades to my grandmother's burial in the Beth Tfiloh cemetery in Baltimore. To bury a loved one is to summon the memories of all the others laid to rest over the years.

My brother, Michael, speaks the truest words:

"Very few people knew my father. I don't mean this in some abstract, philosophical sense. My father was a very private person who had few friends. His life centered around his family. He stubbornly refused to go to any social events. At some point many years ago I realized that the next social event I would be attending with my father would be his funeral.

"Leonard was born in 1919, the last of seven children born to struggling immigrant parents, Jacob and Lizzie. When he was seven years old, his father died, leaving his wife and children to cope with a new business while they did their best to survive the Depression. The experiences and struggles of his youth forged him into the imperfect person that he was. Despite all this, he served his country for almost five years in the Army Air Corps, fell in love and married my mother, re-started and ran a difficult business during difficult times, raised two boys, and did his best to be a good husband, a good father, a loving grandfather, and a good brother to his siblings.

"Besides his family, my dad had many passions in his life. He loved bird-watching and nature, he was an avid fisherman, loved working around his house and his gardens. He rediscovered his artistic gifts later in life and filled the walls of his home with paintings. The subjects of his work were most often his family members.

"My mother was my father's companion of sixty years, his best friend, his great love, the mother of his children, the source of his emotional support, and, in the end, his selfless caregiver. We all did our best these last difficult years, but my mother—more than any of us in our family—refused to give in and place my father into a long-term-care facility. I know I can speak for my father when I say that he was a very lucky man."

When my brother finishes, it is my turn.

"My father was an uneducated man in the formal sense. He never completed high school and he was always ashamed of this, a shame that left him with a crippling inferiority complex and forever on the fringes of social intercourse, and, at times, alienated him even from his own family. As my brother said, he was an imperfect man. But no more or less imperfect than either of his sons, than any man who tries, over a lifetime, to do the right thing but sometimes fails.

"My father always searched, in his own way, for meaning in this life. For many months before his death he carried this copy of Bernard Malamud's book, *God's Grace*, with him wherever he went. It was on his bed beside him when he fell asleep or on his nightstand. He clutched it as one might a talisman even as he tried to negotiate his walker from room to room. Its dust jacket is torn and every page is dog-eared. When I looked for this book last night I found it tucked into the drawer of his nightstand where he kept his special mementoes, cards and letters he had received. This was the only book in the drawer. He had stored it there for safekeeping in case he never got back to it. Now he never will.

"My father struggled, in his way, and mostly alone, to educate himself, to become a fuller person during his lifetime. My brother and I and our families are a testament to his success and his hard-earned wisdom. I pray that he has the blessing of God's Grace from now on."

I end my eulogy by reading a poem by Edward Hirsch.

Lay Back the Darkness

My father in the night shuffling from room to room
on an obscure mission through the hallway.

Help me, spirits, to penetrate his dream
and ease his restless passage.

Lay back the darkness for a salesman
who could charm everything but the shadows,

an immigrant who stands on the threshold
of a vast night

without his walker or his cane
and cannot remember what he meant to say,

though his right arm is raised, as if in prophecy,
while his left shakes uselessly in warning.

My father in the night shuffling from room to room
is no longer a father or a husband or a son,

but a boy standing on the edge of a forest
listening to the distant cry of wolves,

to wild dogs,
to primitive wingbeats shuddering in the treetops.

As his casket slowly descends into the ground, I place my father's copy of *God's Grace* on top of it. Then my brother and I, and everyone present so inclined, shovel the dirt back into that insatiable hole.

The next morning at seven thirty I meet my brother at his synagogue. It is a weekday and only the usual handful of retired men and women—the old old and the oldest old—are there. They recite the morning prayers, make up the *minyen* for the families in mourning, chant the Kaddish, kibitz with each other afterward over coffee and bagels.

My brother hands me a velvet bag containing the tiny boxes, tefillin, that religious Jews attach with leather straps to their forehead and arm each morning during prayers. These boxes contain biblical verses and are the literal manifestation of the command to "bind them as a sign on your head and let them serve as a frontlet between your eyes." I take them from my brother and unzip the bag. But I can't put them on. I am my father's son. I think about my mother sitting alone in her dark house and know what I must do. My brother will have to carry on in the traditional ways without me. I am happy for him that he finds solace in this ritual.

My brother feels strongly that we should maintain a house of mourning—a shiva house—for a few more days, perhaps a week. There we would sit together, think about Dad, deprive ourselves of the routines of daily life in order to focus our thoughts on him, and go to shul morning and night to recite the Kaddish. During these times, traditionally, family and friends come over to the shiva house, and bring food and comfort and support to the family.

But we have no large family. Our friends have already come to the burial and to the house afterward. There will be no more visitors, no more food trays. Just my mother and brother, our wives—neither of them born Jewish—and me. When I offer to take my mother out to the ranch in Comfort, she accepts without hesitation.

After Lee moved to Texas so we could begin our life together, we took weekend drives through the Hill Country just north of San Antonio. We both have grown children, aging parents. Lee had already lost her father. We were starting a new life together, but we had no illusions that it would necessarily be a long one: after all, each of us had already been married twenty-seven years to our first spouses.

We found our small piece of rolling hills and Southern prairie—a rundown, overgrazed ranch, first settled by German Freethinkers one hundred fifty years ago. The graveyards of these early settlers dot the landscape throughout the region. It is here in Comfort, Texas, where we have put down our roots, roots as shallow as the mountain junipers', those thirsty trees trying to grow into the limestone bedrock that lies just inches below the surface of the ground. This is our true home now, and living with nature all around us we both feel that there is nothing "unnatural" about death.

Not far from our place there is a turn-off toward the Guadalupe River. If you take it, the narrow gravel road dips into the bottomland where in the fall, if there has been rain, the fields will wave green with alfalfa, the last crop before winter takes hold. Suddenly you drop down into the riverbed itself: Cypress trees, their fringy leaves now orange, loom overhead on both sides of the quiet banks. The Guadalupe is green and slow and usually at this time of the year it is easy to cross on the low concrete bridge—little more than a fording spot—only inches above the waters of the river. Sometimes—after the spring rains—the river is impassable here; it would swallow us, vehicle and all.

Lee and I always stop near the bridge for a few moments—there is rarely another traveler here—and listen to the wind and water, look up and down the banks. Often we see green kingfishers and great blue herons. We are grateful to be together in this lush and sheltered place. Lee seems to absorb the river's calm. I am ever mindful of that future river, swollen with the rains to come, bearing down.

On the other side of the river, carved out of an alfalfa field, is a small graveyard. It is surrounded by a rusty iron fence and most of it is a tangle of weeds and vines. The headstones are askew; many of them mark tiny graves. There are a few ancient oaks shading this patch of earth from the heat of the Texas sun. It is a family graveyard, tucked into a corner of the family farm. The pioneer homestead had everything, including a final resting place. Nothing seems more natural.

———

On the day after we bury my father, Lee and I pick my mother up and drive the forty miles to the ranch. My mother has not spent a night away from her home in a year and a half—and that was to attend the funeral of her only sister back in Baltimore.

On the way out of town she is silent. It is a magnificent day, the temperature in the seventies. I describe the scenery to her as we drive along. The mountain laurels are beginning to spill their blue blooms and the redbuds are just showing the tiniest pink florets along their bare stems. "Soon it will be spring," I say to her.

My wife and I cook for her. We make up her bed. We drive her around the little town of Comfort, browse the antiques shops, have lunch at the Hen House Café. We watch a couple of movies on TV; if my mother sits very close she can see some of the faces and we fill in with commentary.

She sits quietly for hours looking out the window into the field across from the house. I know she is unable to see any detail. In another month and a half that field will be a profusion of wildflowers. Among the blooms will flit tiger swallowtails, red admirals, and tawny emperors, green darners, and calico pennants. The summer tanager, blue grosbeak, orchard oriole, and scissor-tailed flycatcher will return then, and of course, the indigo buntings. My mother will not see them, but I will tell her.

She does not cry in my presence. When I ask her how she is doing, she will only say, "I keep seeing his face. I keep seeing him lying out there on the lawn."

On the morning before we return to San Antonio, I decide to clean out the purple martin house in anticipation of their arrival. They are the earliest harbingers of spring migration. Martins need a clean place to build their mud-and-stick abodes.

My mother sits in a chair outside the house as Lee and I, ladder in hand, walk across the big field to get the job done. It takes our collective strength to raise the pole up to its full height. By the time we walk back to where my mother sits, a lone male martin has taken his place atop the house, calling for his mates, proclaiming this spot as his own.

"I see why you love this place," my mother says. "It's so peaceful here."

"It's my home now," I say. "When the time comes, I want to be buried here."

"Don't talk about such a thing," she says.

Later in the day, after we clean ourselves up, I ask my mother if she'd like me to read to her from the early manuscript of this book.

"Oh, I would like that," she says.

I read her the chapter I have just completed, the chapter on falling. It reminds her that, despite our best efforts, we were unable to keep my father from falling, about all the things we tried to do to protect him. The words remind her that we thought Dad would likely die from the consequences of a fall and how we would handle it when the time came. I can barely get through the last page or so.

"What do you think?" I say, blowing my nose.

"I just feel so terrible, leaving those keys in the door like I did," she says. Then her tears come. I hold her, tell her that I love her. Over and over I say that she is not to blame, that her guilt will not bring Dad back. Her life, her welfare, her happiness—however much time is left to her—is what is important to my brother and me now.

When we take her home that night, I say that I hope she had a good time in the country.

"It was like medicine for me," she says.

TWENTY-SEVEN

Yesterday my brother and I went to the cemetery to visit our father's grave. A month has passed since his funeral. My brother has been going to synagogue twice daily to recite the Kaddish prayer. His face is fuzzy with an overgrowth of beard. He has spent the last month thinking about our father, about our family now left in the world without him.

After a prolonged South Texas drought, some rains have fallen and the dirt on the top of our father's grave sprouts a few tufts of grass, especially in the center where there is a dip in the ground.

"It shouldn't be this way," my brother says.

"It looks okay to me," I say.

"The dirt should be mounded so that the water runs off the sides and not down into the grave. That pine box won't last very long if it stays wet," he says.

"Mikey, Dad is supposed to return to the earth. That's why we buried him, right?"

He doesn't answer me at first. I put my arm around him. His eyes are brimming.

After a while he says, "I was with him, you know, the evening before he got out of the house . . ."

"I know you were."

"He was very confused and agitated. He kept saying over and
over that he wanted to go home. 'I want to go home,' he said. 'Please
take me home . . .' Mom was beside herself. I stayed a long time and
finally Dad settled down. I even got him to laugh a little . . ."

"Mikey, I know. You called me. I told you to search through
Dad's medicines. In the basket up in the kitchen cabinets, remember?
I told you to find the risperidone and give him one and you did.
That's why he finally settled down . . ."

My brother is crying now. I hold him in my arms, my little
brother who has been taller than I since I can't remember when. His
sobs shake my body.

"I should have slept there that night. I thought about doing it. I
would have been right there on the living room couch and I would
have heard him get up that morning."

I push my brother back so I can look into his face. He has my father's gray eyes.

"Listen to me, Mikey. What if he hadn't died that morning? Then
what?"

Guilt is so powerful, so destructive. It's bred into most of us from
an early age. I have no easy answers about guilt. I have borne my
share, more than my share. I still bear it: guilt about how I have lived
my life as a son, as a husband, as a father. And, of course, as a doctor.

Now that my father is in the ground, now that some time has
passed, now that it is clear that my mother, even rested and unbur-
dened with daily caregiving, is rapidly approaching the point where
she will need the kind of attention my father received in his last
years, it is time for me to grapple with the guilt I feel as his son.

Could I have been a better doctor to my father? This may sound
like a strange question. After all, I was not my father's doctor of record.
It was not I who admitted him to the hospital six years ago when he
descended into delirium. I did not see him for his follow-up visits

every few months. I did not prescribe his medications, send him for consultations, order his laboratory testing. I was not the doctor who signed his death certificate.

Yet I was heavily involved in my father's medical care. How could I not be? How could his son, the geriatrician, the one visiting several times a week, sometimes daily, the family member who has spent a life observing the effects of the aging process on thousands of people, their responses to medications, the one able to spot a change in his patient instantly upon walking into an exam room—how could I not be involved in my father's care? How could I fail to notice when he was more short of breath and could do with a bit more diuretic? Or hear my mother's concerns about his agitation or anxiety or nighttime perambulations and not try a slight dosage change in the medications used to control these behaviors?

Dr. William Osler, the father of Internal Medicine, once said that the physician who treats himself has a fool for a patient. Perhaps, by extension, I was a fool to treat my own father at times.

On the night in question, the night before the morning my father eloped into the backyard of his home and died, the night my brother called me to report that Dad was more confused and agitated than usual, that he could not rest, that he just "wanted to go home," I made a decision over the phone—a medical decision—to treat my father with a dose of risperidone. This was an antipsychotic medication that my father had taken before, prescribed by his physician, in tiny doses, and with good success. My father needed this drug only rarely and I knew that there was an almost-full bottle of it in a basket of medications on the top shelf of the kitchen cabinet above the sink.

"Give him one risperidone pill," I told my brother when he called me that night. Who should know better than me: the older brother, the geriatrician, the devoted and loving son?

There are things I did not tell my brother that night. I did not tell him that my father's increased agitation constituted a "condition change." This is a term that medical practitioners in the long-term-care field use to describe any acute change in the status of a patient.

A condition change might be something obvious—a patient who spikes a temperature to 101 degrees, for example. But many of these changes are subtler—an elderly woman who begins to fall more of-ten, a man who suddenly has several episodes of urinary incontinence, a patient whose speech becomes slurred. Sometimes a condition change might be a behavioral one—a new tendency toward bel-ligerency, a recent penchant for insomnia, falling asleep during meal-time. Or an increase in agitation.

If I had a patient like my father in a long-term-care facility I would expect a call from the nursing staff to alert me to any significant condi-tion change. The staff, of course, is expected to provide me with as much information as they can: any physical complaint my patient might have, her temperature and blood pressure and pulse rate; any physical signs the staff might notice—a cough, new bruises, or foul-smelling urine, for instance. I would ask about my patient's eating habits, ability to swallow, the integrity of her skin, her recent bowel movements. I would review the medication list.

Then I would have to make a decision, requiring much judgment but always fraught with peril. Can we watch and wait and see what happens by tomorrow? Do I need to come in tonight and examine the patient myself? Should I send this confused, elderly person into the tumult of the emergency room, an experience that will cost thou-sands of dollars, and only create fear and havoc in the mind of my patient?

Or do I, with all the information I have collected from the facil-ity staff, knowing it is incomplete, prescribe something that may just help, may avoid a crisis, may settle the patient down, get her through the night—that time when so many of the aged experience an in-crease in agitation and confusion?

So this geriatrician-son made a decision, over the phone, based on his extensive past knowledge of his "non-patient," but with a dearth of present information, to try something that had worked in the past. My brother dutifully gave our father 0.5 milligrams of risperidone, just as I told him to do.

I assumed that my father's condition change was due to the usual ups and downs of his underlying dementia. But I asked for no data to the contrary. Where was I to get it? I was in Comfort that night, not just down the street. I thought about sending my father into the emergency room, but this was something I had promised him and my family I would never do again.

And so I reached for a pharmacological solution to the problem.

There was something else I did not tell my brother when he sobbed in my arms at the edge of the grave awash in guilt, that I did not tell my mother as she has suffered with her own guilt this last month over leaving her key dangling in the kitchen door.

It might have been the risperidone that killed my father.

A few months before my father's death the FDA placed a "black box" warning label on risperidone and on all the so-called atypical antipsychotic medications that have become so popular in the treatment of behavorial and psychotic disturbances in our demented elderly patients. The warning reads:

> *Elderly patients with dementia-related psychosis treated with atypical anti-psychotic drugs are at an increased risk of death compared to placebo . . . most of the deaths appeared to be either cardiovascular . . . or infectious . . . in nature.* **Risperidone is not approved for the treatment of patients with dementia-related psychosis.**

I knew all of this, of course. I decided to use risperidone because it had worked before and it was right there in the kitchen. When I think rationally about it, do I believe that the single dose I had my brother administer to my father was the cause of his death? No, I don't. More to the point, would I use this drug again for my father under similar circumstances? Yes. But what about for your mother or your father or your spouse? We would talk about it, weigh the pros and cons, the risks and benefits—and the decision would be yours, assuming you have the legal authority to make it. That is what I as a

geriatrician bring to you, the family of an aging, debilitated, and demented loved one: compassion and judgment and experience. Not
perfection.

I made a medical decision the night my brother called me. I think
it was the right decision—and many geriatric experts would side
with me and not the FDA. Still, this does not mean that I don't have
any guilt about it. Guilt—especially over medical decisions—is, by
now, annealed to my bones. Of course, my mother and brother won't
bring a malpractice suit against me. So why even bring this up?

We are all children of aging parents, spouses or caregivers to
loved ones at the end of their lives. Or we will be. Or we were. I
have spent my life as a doctor endeavoring to do the best job I could
do. I was never perfect; on occasion I failed. I always learned from
my mistakes, but I continue to live with them.

I loved my father, an imperfect and often difficult man. It was
understood in my family that I would be the one to make the medical decisions on his behalf when he became unable to do so. He was
not the kind of man who would ever talk about what he wanted at
life's end. In the years before his dementia took hold, if I tried to
engage him about his wishes on the subjects of cardio-pulmonary
resuscitation or ventilators or tube-feedings, he would wave me off
with his hand. *What do you want to talk about that depressing stuff for?*
he would say, or, *What, you can't wait?* These conversations went
nowhere or opened old wounds. A number of years before he died,
before his dementia, my father did designate me—in writing—as his
legal surrogate decision-maker. I dropped off the papers one night,
asked my parents to look them over and sign them. Without fanfare,
without further questions, they did. And when the time came, I
made the decisions. And still there is guilt.

If I have it, chances are you do, too. You are there alone in the
house with your debilitated or demented loved one. You have flown
in from across the continent and are now at the bedside of your father or mother in a hospital ICU, wondering what to do next as the
respirator hisses and clicks in the corner. You pace the halls of the

nursing home as the aides finally come to clean the excrement from your mother's bottom, apply the protective unguents to the inflamed flesh. Or you sit again at a bedside, watching as a bag of opaque liquid is pumped, drop by drop, through the plastic tubing which snakes under the sheets and into the stomach of someone you once knew and still love.

You feel guilty and powerless and abandoned and angry and bereft. You have decisions to make and no one to guide you. Your father's doctor or some anonymous "care team" on daily rounds floats in and out of the room very early or very late. You think they are trying to avoid you on purpose, your difficult questions. And maybe they are. Your own children live far away. Your siblings are obstinate or in denial or still angry over some long ago slight, some falling out which seems silly now.

You are afraid that you will make a mistake, decide the wrong thing, choose the wrong path. *Honor thy father and thy mother.* Your head spins: *Oh God, how can I not feed her through this tube? If I demand it be removed, if I discontinue this infernal respirator I know he will die. The doctor says she must go back into the hospital to treat this pneumonia. Again. How many times can she survive this? Is this hurting him? Would she want this? If I say, "Enough!" am I committing a sin? Murder? Will Mom forgive me? My sister? Will I ever be able to forgive myself?*

If you are the family of one of my patients and we are facing a difficult situation, an end-of-life scenario so common in the geriatric setting, we will sit down together and talk. I will answer all of your questions truthfully as I see the situation at that moment. I will present options; nothing need be written in stone. Any decisions made can be changed up until the last moment.

If you ask me what I would do if this were my father or my mother or my wife, I will tell you, if I know. For me to answer this question for you—in this age when the precept of patient autonomy rules over the principle of beneficence—might be considered paternalistic by some. I have helped too many folks through difficult times to be dissuaded by the thought that I may be offending the ethical sensibilities of some who might second-guess me from afar.

Ultimately, however, the decision will be yours. And I will respect it even if I disagree as long as you do not ask me to commit malpractice or perform an illegal act. As long as I have your respect and your confidence, we will continue to muddle through together. And "the end will come in its time," as Dr. William Carlos Williams once wrote.

If I failed my father, if I bear some measure of guilt as his son, it is not over the decisions I made the night before he died or for my care the last years of his life when his dementia became obvious to us all and I did my best to keep him at home and comfortable. I have no guilt over making any decision that may have favored the quality of his life over the quantity of it.

Still, I could have been a better son. Who understood his foibles, his failings better than I, his oldest son and the inheritor of many of his personality traits, for better or worse? I understood, but I was, for too many years, unable to forgive my father his failings. Somehow I expected him to overcome his lack of self-esteem, his limited education and insular upbringing, rise above his misfortune and bad luck, and make a new life for himself after he lost the only business he knew at age fifty—only ten years younger than I am now. He was unable to do it—how many among us could?—and I know that too often I let my disappointment in him show.

I have heard psychologists say that each of us is responsible for the happiness of only one person, and that person is ourself. I do believe that this is true even though it has taken me, a caregiver forged by nature and nurture, most of my life to strike a proper balance.

And yet when our parents become old and feeble we are responsible for them, are we not? Are we not responsible for our children when they are small and vulnerable in the wider world? I am not equating our elderly with children—they should not be thought of or treated as such. But we—our society, and ultimately our families—are responsible for our frail aged, for their well-being, for continuing to show them love, valuing them so that they will, in turn, still feel valuable. This is a family matter, not a state matter, not a policy issue or a legal conundrum.

Of course these societal problems deserve good public policymaking by knowledgeable and compassionate people. We must, as a nation, realize that very soon well over a million people will have no living spouse or siblings or children and many millions of others will lack the means to secure a safe and dignified old age. But policy matters aside, we must come together as families, friends, and neighbors and do what it takes to ensure that our elders receive respect and compassion in their waning years.

When it is finally your husband's or wife's, or your mother's or father's time to go, when the heart monitor falls silent, the respirator ceases with a sigh, the hum of the feeding pump fades away, the chest settles for the last time, you will, most likely, feel some measure of guilt. You will wonder if you gave up the fight too soon. Or perhaps you hung in there, bruised and bleeding, another round or two almost beyond your endurance. You may be disappointed in the health-care system, your doctor, the hospital, the nursing home. You may want to blame someone, some institution—and there is, unfortunately, usually plenty of blame to go around.

But bearing this guilt, carrying this anger will not ease any suffering, will not bring your loved one back, will not help you heal, and will not prepare you for the next loss, the next ordeal which is coming. Devote whatever energies you can muster to being kinder, more understanding, more loving to those who are still on this earth and to whom you are still responsible. And save some for yourself, because you will need it.

I must quote my father here, his words that come back to me

now, words meant to make me a better person in this world, boost me beyond—if not my own yearnings and capabilities to succeed, then at least his.

Here is what he would say: *Let that be a lesson to you.*

I wish that my father, my brother, and I had taken more trips together to the Texas coast, especially in the springtime, when wave upon wave of migrating flocks of orioles and tanagers and buntings and warblers brave the uncertainties of a nighttime passage over the Gulf to find themselves, breathless in the morning light, sheltered in the coastal live oak groves of the Central Flyway. My father was the closest he ever came to happiness when we were all together, standing side by side in the high grass on Live Oak Point, among the thousand-year-old trees, the rising sun glinting off the waters of Aransas Bay, the taste of salt-spray on our lips, our binoculars fixed on a rose-breasted grosbeak—his chest pink as a sunset, his head black as a moonless night—watching him hop from limb to limb, forage just a few arm-lengths away.

"Over here!" my father calls to me.

"I see him, Dad! He's magnificent . . ."

"You'll remember this for the rest of your life, won't you, Jerry-boy?"

TWENTY-EIGHT

A year is a small piece in the life of a man. Yet so much can happen, so much can change. Almost every week one of my old friends passes on. In this year I said good-bye to Mrs. Ash who, at ninety-one, finally succumbed to her lung cancer after a six-year battle. Mr. Casey had one last stroke that took him, mercifully quickly, at eighty-eight. Mrs. Brown, eighty-four, fell at home, couldn't get up, lay on the floor for two days before anyone came looking for her. By the time we got her to the hospital she was in kidney failure and didn't survive. Every week it is like this.

My father has been gone a year now and during this time I have been working on this book and thinking about him, about his life, about my life as his son. When I began my book in the fall of 2005, I imagined him leafing through its pages, even though I knew for certain that whatever he read—if he could still read—would be forgotten in the next instant. I can hear him asking me: *Did you really write all this yourself?*

My mother lives on in their home. Yolanda comes almost every day, and my brother and I and our wives are in and out constantly.

Mom's vision continues to worsen; we must guard her on any outing we take, keep an arm extended for her to hold. She has fallen in the house several times, thankfully without serious injury. She won't hear of an assisted-living facility.

We have just returned from the cemetery for the ceremony that Jews call the "unveiling." My brother had a simple footstone carved and placed at the gravesite. It says only, LEONARD WINAKUR, 2/1/19–2/28/06, BELOVED HUSBAND, FATHER, AND GRANDFATHER. Just a few words— but perhaps this is more than enough for one lifetime. My brother and I chanted the Kaddish together once again.

For months we have been urging my mother to begin the process of sorting through my father's things. Now she seems ready. Her Baltimore cousins, Rita and Buddy, are coming for a visit in a few weeks and will stay in the house, sleep in my father's bedroom, her first guests in many years. She is ready for this, rested now that the daily burden of my father's care has been lifted.

A week after the unveiling, one evening after work, I stop by to see my mother. It is time to refill her pill containers for the next month.

"Go into Dad's bedroom and take whatever you want," she says. "Next week Yolanda and I will bag up the rest and give it to Goodwill."

I have avoided my father's room this past year. Whenever I did walk in, I expected to see him lying in his bed, a book by his side. When he wasn't there, a lump rose in my throat. The hospital bed is gone now and the old marital bed is back in its place, flanked by the two end tables. The bookcases, still full, stand along one wall.

I open my father's closet. I am overwhelmed with the smell of him—his Old Spice, his deodorant, his sweat. The closet is packed with decades of his clothing, some in mint condition—the blue serge suit he wore to my Bar Mitzvah, the black pinstripe to my first wedding. All his rayon fishing shirts hang in a row. His older clothes are too big for me, the newer ones too small. It seems we were never the same size. Way in the back is an old corduroy shirt covered with blue and green and white paint spatters. This is the shirt he wore in his garage studio on winter days as he feverishly worked over a canvas. I pull it from its hanger.

His old Army binoculars sit on the top shelf. Long ago I had returned these to him; I bought myself a new pair—stronger magnification, greater depth of field, brighter image. I finger the old leather strap, now cracked and frayed; I put the glasses around my neck. The lenses are coated with dust, but they will clean up easily. Seen through these, the birds will appear smaller, a bit less bright, but they will come into focus just the same. And the glasses feel very light in my hands.

I open the bottom drawer of my father's dresser. This is where my mother stowed his pajamas. They are still here along with the workout pants and shirts he wore the last several years of his life. These uniforms of the oldest old are folded neatly, ready to be worn again after having been laundered and bleached by my mother. Even so, there are stains on the pants. When I bring the pile to my face and close my eyes, he is here.

I slide them all into a shopping bag. Most are too small for me. At least for now. I will take them out to Comfort and put them away. One day—if I make it as many years as my Dad—I will wear these uniforms of my father's oldest days as I shuffle into my own. I will wrap myself in his smells and no doubt add my own before it is over. I will feel him around me. I will be him.

I want to remember.

ACKNOWLEDGMENTS

Without my patients this book would not exist. Whatever I have learned about the human condition I have learned from them. We have listened to each other; we have come to know one another; we have grown old together. They are my surrogate family. They have enriched my life beyond my imaginings.

I am grateful to my family of origin. We have had our share of ups and downs and certainly these last years have been very trying. My father's love, my mother's perseverance, my brother, Michael's, steadiness and support have all helped me through these times as well as through my life.

My devoted daughters, Betsy and Emily—both strong, accomplished women now—have been a source of great pride to me. Their insights and their love have informed this book. Their mother, Dr. Leslie Winakur, my first wife, will forever have my admiration and affection. We grew up together in medicine, became better doctors because of what we learned from each other, shared our mutual triumphs and failures. I could not have been successful had she not been by my side in medical school, residency, and our years of practice.

There are other members of my family who deserve mention. My cousin, Dr. Charles Merrill, has provided me with invaluable encouragement, help, and reference materials. Stan and Cindy Merrill have given me considerable moral and technical support. Another cousin, Mr. Herbert Dunn, has been a comfort and friend to his uncle, my father, as well as to the rest of my family.

Dan and Chaddie Kruger have been good friends through the years.

I have had many wonderful mentors along the way. Professor Michael Rosenzweig and his wife Carole at Bucknell University, Dr. Edward Stemmler at the University of Pennsylvania School of Medicine, Dr. Marvin Forland at the University of Texas Health Science Center at San Antonio.

In my life as a practicing physician, I am grateful for the assistance and dedication of four women over these last thirty-plus years: Anna Talamantes, Frances Winakur, Isabella Cantu, and Alyson Guerrero. Without them, loyal and earnest in their work, my patients would not have been so well cared for.

I am grateful to Dr. John Galan who, with patience and wisdom, cared for my parents in their old old years, and to Dr. Hoan Pho, my own personal physician.

My first writing mentor—professor emeritus at Trinity University here in San Antonio—is and remains Eugene McKinney. His early encouragement was instrumental in my continued attempts to write and I am grateful for his friendship—and for that of his wife, Treysa—and for their feedback on an early draft of this book.

There are so many others who have helped and encouraged me: Professor Wendy Barker at the University of Texas at San Antonio; Wayne Johnson at the Iowa Summer Writer's Workshop; the poet Maxine Kumin and her husband, Victor; Cheri Peters at the Sewanee Writer's Conference; Alan Shapiro at Bread Loaf.

Special thanks to Dr. Abraham Verghese and the other members of our Physicians Writing Group at the Center for Medical Humanities and Ethics here at the UTHSCSA, where the original essay that became this book was presented.

I am also grateful to Dr. Therese Jones at the University of Utah Health Science Center for her friendship and for her guidance in the field of Medical Humanities. I also want to thank Dean Daniel Gelo at the University of Texas at San Antonio and Dean Michael Fischer at Trinity University for giving my wife, Lee Robinson, and me the opportunity to teach our Medical Humanities and Ethics courses to their undergraduates.

The physician-writer Dr. Gene Radice published some of my earliest work in his magazine, *Mediphors—A Literary Journal of the Health Professions*. My experience as a contributing editor to this periodical that gave voice to so many medical professionals was a formative one.

I am indebted to Ellen Ficklen and Fitzhugh Mullan of *Health Affairs* for selecting my essay, "What Are We Going to Do with Dad?," for inclusion in the "Narrative Matters" section of this publication, and to the *Washington Post* for their excerpt of this piece that gave it such wide attention.

Thanks are also due to Carolyn Banks for the opportunity to author a monthly column, "Meditations on Medicine," in the journal *LifeTimes*, published by Blue Cross Blue Shield. Her confidence in my writing allowed me to first explore some of the ideas for this book, and her editing has only improved my efforts.

I have been privileged to be a part of San Antonio's own nonprofit literary organization, Gemini Ink, these last ten years. It has been a joy to watch this endeavor—begun by Nan Cuba—grow under the directorship of Rose Catacalos into an important force for the literary arts and literacy in my city. I have been enlightened—as have so many of my fellow citizens—by the international talent that has come to San Antonio through the efforts of Gemini Ink, even as we continue to nurture our own.

I must also thank the editor of Trinity University Press, the poet Barbara Ras, for her early encouragement of this manuscript.

You would not be holding this book were it not for the faith placed in me by my agent, Mary Evans or by my editor at Hyperion, Brenda Copeland. I will always be grateful to both of them.

For ten years my life has been enriched by my best friend, my first reader and demanding editor—my wife, the lawyer-poet Lee Robinson. This book has been enhanced and its writing clarified by her efforts; the faults that remain are entirely mine. Whatever life and time have in store for us as we enter our "Golden Years," thanks to Lee I have already had mine.

Jonah Leo Tontiplaphol, born ten months after the death of my father, will never know this great-grandfather. One day, I hope that this book with its secondhand stories will teach my grandson some important lessons so that Great-Grandpa Leonard might live on in Jonah's own memories.

Portions of this book have appeared in earlier and different versions in the following publications: *Health Affairs, Life Times, Penn Medicine, Mediphors—A Literary Journal of the Health Professions, The New Physician,* and *Chesapeake Bay.*

"Creed," by Lee Robinson, first appeared in *Kalliope.*

NOTES

INTRODUCTION

2   *I wrote an essay*: Winakur, Jerald, "What Are We Going to Do with Dad?", *Health Affairs,* July/August 2005, Vol. 24, No. 4, pp.1064–72.

3   *Today there are 4.5 million people*: *Taking Care: Ethical Caregiving in Our Aging Society,* The President's Council on Bioethics, September 2005.

3   *By 2030 there will be seventy-two million people*: Ibid.

ONE

8   *Seventy-five percent of Americans*: Henig, Robin M., "Will We Ever Arrive at the Good Death?", *New York Times Magazine,* August 7, 2005.

FOUR

40   *one recent survey*: Croasdale, Myrle, "Lack of supervision adds to resident errors, study finds," *American Medical News,* November 26, 2007.

41   *the story of Dax Cowart*: *Please Let Me Die,* Robert B. White, Director, University of Texas Medical Branch, Galveston, Texas, 1974.

42 *the movie* Wit: *Wit,* A Film by Mike Nichols, HBO, 2001.

42 *The status of health care: Code Red: The Critical Condition of Health Care in Texas,* a report of the Task Force on Access to Health Care in Texas, April 17, 2006 (see full report at www.CodeRedTexas.org).

FIVE

57 *multi-generational households*: Navarro, Mireya, "Families Add Third Generation to Households," *New York Times,* May 25, 2006.

SIX

60 *Geriatrics is very much*: Gross, Jane, "Geriatrics Lags in Age of High-Tech Medicine," *New York Times,* October 18, 2006.

61 *Dr. Eric Cassel notes*: Cassel, Eric J., "The Nature of Suffering and the Goals of Medicine," *New England Journal of Medicine,* Vol. 306, No. 11, 1982.

65 *an oversupply of specialists*: Schneider, Mary Ellen, "ACP Charts New Path for Internists," *Internal Medicine News,* May 2006, Vol. 39, Issue 9, p. 1.

67 *a recent study has shown*: Farber, Jeffrey, et al., "How Much Time Do Physicians Spend Providing Care Outside of Office Visits?", *Annals of Internal Medicine,* November 20, 2007, Vol. 47, No. 10, pp. 693–98.

67 *the overall cost*: Weiss, L. J., et al., "Faithful patients: The Effect of Long-term Physician-patient Relationships on the Costs and Use of Health Care by Older Americans," *American Journal of Public Health,* 1996, 86(12):1742–47.

68 *"comprehensive follow-up visit"*: Zuckerman, M. S., et al., "Use of Physician's Services Under Medicare's Resource-based Payments," *New England Journal of Medicine,* 2007, 356: 1853–61.

68 *a fixed payment*: Stone, Dennis, and Tarnove, Elaine, "CPT Codes: The Evolution and Current State of Codes and Their Use," *Journal of the American Medical Directors Association,* November 2001, Vol. 2, Issue 6, pp. 310–14.

68   *Primary care doctors*: Goodson, J. D., "Unintended Consequences of Resource-Based Value Scale Reimbursement," *Journal of the American Medical Association*, November 21, 2007, 298(19): 2308–10.

68   *"current reimbursement incentives"*: Based on Medicare's Current Procedural Terminology Fee Schedule, 2005.

69   *And over 90 percent*: Goodson, op. cit.

69   *in unprecedented numbers*: Croasdale, M., "Record Number Vied for Medical School Slots," *American Medical News*, November 5, 2007, Vol. 50, No. 41, p. 1.

70   *They want to do it*: Schneider, op. cit.

70   *about three hundred*: "Statement on Patients in Peril: Critical Shortages in Geriatric Care," *The Association of American Medical Colleges* Statement to the Special Committee on Aging, United States Senate, March 13, 2002, p. 3.

SEVEN

76   *will be above average*: Garibaldi, R. A., "Career Plans for Trainees in Internal Medicine Residency Programs," *Academic Medicine*, 2005, 80:507–12.

EIGHT

84   *"non-patients"*: American Medical Association, E-8.19: *Self-Treatment or Treatment of Immediate Family Members;* http://www.ama-assn.org/ama/pub/category/8510.html.

84   *There is survey data*: Latessa and Ray, "Should You Treat Yourself, Family or Friends?", *Family Practice Management,* March 2005.

NINE

93   *even moderate cases*: Solomon, Paul R., et al., "Should We Screen for Alzheimer's Disease?", *Geriatrics*, November 2005, Vol. 60, No. 11, pp. 26–31.

TEN

102   *heard the stories*: Campbell, E. G., et al., "Institutional Academic-Industry
       Relationships," *Journal of the American Medical Association*, October 17,
       2007, Vol. 28, No. 15, pp. 1779–86.

104   *"I lost myself"*: Williams, W. C., *The Autobiography of William Carlos
       Williams*, Random House, New York, 1951, p. 356.

ELEVEN

109   *A conservative estimate*: Shenk, David, "The Memory Hole," *New York
       Times*, November 3, 2006.

110   *variations in clinical patterns*: Brayne, Carol, et al., "Dementia Screening in
       Primary Care: Is It Time?", *Journal of the American Medical Association*,
       November 28, 2007, Vol. 298, No. 20, pp. 2409–11.

110   *standardized mental status testing*: Folstein, M. F., et al., "Mini-Mental
       State: A Practical Method for Grading the Cognitive State of Patients
       for the Clinician, *Journal of Psychiatric Research*, 1975, 12(3): 189–98.

111   Brayne, op. cit.

111   *its earliest stages?*: Solomon, Paul R., et al., "Should We Screen for
       Alzheimer's Disease?", *Geriatrics*, November 2005, Vol. 60, No. 11, pp.
       26–31.

112   *Memantine blocks*: Winblade, et al., "Memantine in Severe Dementia,"
       International Journal of Geriatric Psychiatry, 1999, 14: 135–146.

TWELVE

119   *Nearly twenty Americans*: Cohen, Donna, "Homicide-Suicide in Older
       Persons: How You Can Help Prevent a Tragedy," Department of Aging
       and Mental Health, *The Louis de la Parte Florida Mental Health Institute*,
       University of South Florida, 2001.

FOURTEEN

132   *in her book*: Kumin, Maxine, *Inside the Halo and Beyond: The Anatomy of a Recovery*, W. W. Norton, 2000.

132   Ibid., pp. 155–56.

133   Ibid., p.157.

134   *a landmark article*: Quill, Timothy, "Death and Dignity: A Case of Individualized Decision Making," *New England Journal of Medicine*, March 7, 1991, Vol. 324, No. 10, pp. 691–94.

134   *exactly this scenario*: Death with Dignity Act, Oregon Revised Statutes, 127.800–127.897.

135   *In her book*: Johnson, Harriet M., *Too Late To Die Young: Nearly True Tales from a Life*, Henry Holt, New York, 2005.

135   *in America today*: *Taking Care: Ethical Caregiving in Our Aging Society*, The President's Council on Bioethics, September 2005.

FIFTEEN

138   *Acute hospitalizations*: Gibbs, N., and Bower, A., "What Scares Doctors: What Insiders Know About Our Health-Care System that the Rest of Us Need to Learn," *TIME*, May 1, 2006, pp. 43–52.

141   *spouses constitute*: *Taking Care*, op. cit.

142   *what is the definition*: Saliba, Debra, et al., "Quality Indicators for the Management of Medical Conditions in Nursing Home Residents," *Journal of the American Medical Directors Association*, May/June 2005, pp. 536–48.

143   *studies have shown*: Thomas and Osterweil, "Is a Pressure Ulcer a Marker for Quality of Care?", *Journal of the American Medical Directors Association*, May/June 2005, pp. 228–30.

144   *futurist gurus*: Kurzweil, Ray, *The Singularity Is Near: When Humans Transcend Biology*, Viking, 2005.

144   *the price tag*: Rosofsky, Ira, "Escape from the Nursing Home," *New York Times*, January 17, 2007.

145   *Homesharing*: www.homeshare.org.

145   *another interesting idea*: Basler, B. "Assisted Living: 10 Great Ideas," *AARP Bulletin*, February 2006.

146   *(NORCs)*: Basler, B., "Declaration of Independents," *AARP Bulletin*, December 2005.

146   *Beacon Hill Village*: Gross, Jane, "Aging at Home: For a Lucky Few, a Wish Come True," *New York Times*, February 9, 2006.

146   *an RV park*: Gross, Jane, "A Grass-Roots Effort to Grow Old at Home," *New York Times*, August 14, 2007.

147   Basler, B., *AARP Bulletin*, February 2006, op. cit., p. 22.

147   Ibid., p. 21.

147   *Imprimis*, Hillsdale College, November 2005, 34(11), p. 5, re: Independence Grove.

SIXTEEN

157   *"long-term-care insurance"?*: Duhigg, Charles, "Aged, Frail and Denied by Their Insurers," *New York Times*, March 26, 2007.

157   *Several states*: Curran, John, "Experiment Sends Fewer to Nursing Homes: Vermont Project Saves Money by Paying Kin, Friends as Caregivers," *San Antonio Express-News*, November 2, 2006, p. 9A.

157   *Lawsuits have been filed*: "Laguna Honda Residents Sue San Francisco for Discrimination," AARP Foundation Litigation, *Bazelon Center for Mental Health Law*, Disability Rights Education and Defense Fund, October 13, 2006.

158   *hospitals so dependent*: Dewan, S., et al., "A Safety Net Hospital Falls into Financial Crisis," *New York Times*, January 8, 2008.

158   *Health-care workers*: www.FoxNews.com quoting an AP release, "Food Servers, Personal Care Workers Suffer High Rates of Depression," October 14, 2007.

158   *One million RNs*: www.CodeRedTexas.org., op. cit.

159   *average annual cost*: Ibid.

159   *an efficient system*: Woolhandler, et al., "The Cost of Health Care Administration in the United States and Canada," *New England Journal of Medicine*, 2003, 349:768–75.

SEVENTEEN

165   *a tattered copy*: Malamud, Bernard, *God's Grace*, Farrar, Straus & Giroux, 1982, p. 7.

EIGHTEEN

167   *upon his book*: Piatt, Jean, *Adventures in Birding: Confessions of a Lister*, Knopf, New York, 1973, p. 265.

170   *In his book*: Verghese, Abraham, *The Tennis Partner: A Doctor's Story of Friendship and Loss*, HarperCollins, 1998, p. 341.

TWENTY

180   *Doctors are human*: Groopman, Jerome, "What's the Trouble?" *The New Yorker*, January 29, 2007, p. 38.

183   *The School Sisters*: Snowdon, David, *Aging with Grace: What The Nun Study Teaches Us About Leading Longer, Healthier, and More Meaningful Lives*, Bantam, 2002.

183   Ibid., p. 15.

183   Ibid., pp. 202–3.

185   *the most educated generation*: "Census Foresees an Older, and Wiser, America," *Washington Post*, March 10, 2006.

185   *We should be healthier.* Lyman, Rick, "Census Report Foresees No Crisis over Aging Generation's Health," *New York Times*, March 10, 2006.

TWENTY-ONE

198   *One in three*: Stevens, J. A., et al., "The costs of fatal and non-fatal falls among older adults," *Injury Prevention*, 2006, 12:290-5.

TWENTY-TWO

209   *The FDA has pulled*: Vedantam, Shankar, "FDA Told U.S. Drug System Is Broken," *Washington Post*, September 23, 2006.

209   *He took Vioxx*: Kaufman, Marc, "Merck Found Liable in Vioxx Case," *Washington Post*, August 20, 2005.

210   *Now that they*: Angell, M., "Your Dangerous Drugstore," *New York Review of Books*, June 8, 2006, pp. 38–40.

211   *any physician who prescribes*: "Atypical Antipsychotics and the Geriatric Patient: Balancing Safety and Efficacy," *Geriatrics*, July 2007, pp. 12, 15.

211   *Medications like risperidone*: Campbell, E. G., op. cit.

211   *the money they receive*: Elliott, Carl, "Guinea-pigging," *The New Yorker*, January 7, 2008, pp. 36–41.

216   *many spousal caregivers*: Kornblum, Janet, "Caregiver's health in 'downward spiral,'" *USA Today*, September 24, 2006.

TWENTY-THREE

225   *End-of-life medical care*: *Center to Advance Palliative Care Manual*, Center to Advance Palliative Care, New York, NY, 2001.

232   *unneeded suffering*: "[There is] no direct data to support tube feeding of demented patients with eating difficulties for any of the commonly cited indications. Tube feeding is a risk factor for aspiration pneumonia. . . . Survival has not shown to be prolonged. Feeding tubes have not been shown to improve pressure sore outcomes, and in fact, the relationship between nutrient intake and pressure sores is tenuous at best . . . [and

tubes have] not been shown to reduce infection. Functional status has not been improved and demented patients are not made more comfortable with tube feeding while dozens of serious adverse effects have been reported."

Finucane, T. E., et al., "Tube Feeding in Patients with Advanced Dementia: A Review of the Evidence," *Journal of the American Medical Association*, October 13, 1999, 282:1365–70.

TWENTY-FOUR

239   *Advance Directives*: Kass, Leon, "Lingering Longer: Who Will Care?" *New York Times*, September 29, 2005, p. A23.

TWENTY-FIVE

246   *Families of the oldest*: Benkendorf, et al., "Outcomes of Cardiac Arrest in the Nursing Home: Destiny or Futility?" *Prehospital Emergency Care*, 1997, 1:68–72.

TWENTY-SIX

257   Hirsch, Edward, "Lay Back the Darkness," from *Lay Back the Darkness*, Knopf, New York, 2003.

TWENTY-SEVEN

266   *the FDA placed*: Risperidone, FDA black-box warning label, *Physicians' Desk Reference 2006*, p. 1660.

266   *and on all the so-called*: "Atypical Antipsychotics and the Geriatric Patient: Balancing Safety and Efficacy," *Geriatrics*, July 2007, p.16.

269   *"the end will come"*: Williams, William Carlos, "Asphodel, That Greeny Flower," from *The Collected Poems of William Carlos Williams*, New Directions (1991), Vol. 2, 1939–62, p. 310.

269   *we are responsible*: *Taking Care*, op. cit.